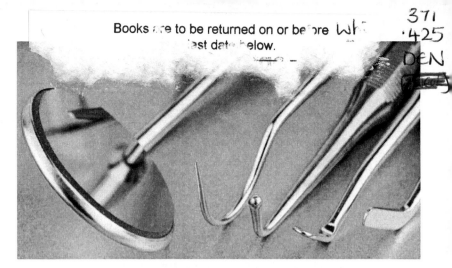

Succeeding in your Application to Dental School

How to prepare the perfect UCAS statement

Matt Gr...

D0552247

BPP

LEARNING MEDIA

First edition September 2011

ISBN 9781 4453 7963 0

British Library Cataloguing-in-Publication Data
A catalogue record for this book is available from
the British Library

Published by
BPP Learning Media Ltd
BPP House, Aldine Place
London W12 8AA

www.bpp.com/health

Typeset by Replika Press Pvt Ltd, India
Printed in the United Kingdom

The views expressed in this book are those of
BPP Learning Media and not those of UCAS. BPP
Learning Media are in no way associated with or
endorsed by UCAS.

The contents of this book are intended as a guide
and not professional advice. Although every effort
has been made to ensure that the contents of
this book are correct at the time of going to
press, BPP Learning Media, the Editor and the
Author make no warranty that the information
in this book is accurate or complete and accept
no liability for any loss or damage suffered by
any person acting or refraining from acting as a
result of the material in this book.

Every effort has been made to contact the
copyright holders of any material reproduced
within this publication. If any have been
inadvertently overlooked, BPP Learning Media
will be pleased to make the appropriate credits
in any subsequent reprints or editions.

Contents

Contents

About the Publisher

BPP Learning Media is dedicated to supporting aspiring professionals with top quality learning material. BPP Learning Media's commitment to success is shown by our record of quality, innovation and market leadership in paper-based and e-learning materials. BPP Learning Media's study materials are written by professionally-qualified specialists who know from personal experience the importance of top quality materials for success.

About the Author

Matt Green BSc (Hons) MPhil

Matt Green has spent the last six years directly helping tens of thousands of individuals successfully apply to university. It is with this extensive experience in mind that Matt has written this book to help applicants prepare an effective UCAS Personal Statement as part of their application to university.

v

Acknowledgements

I would like to thank all of the prospective university students I have supported in the past six years; they have enabled the writing of this book to become a reality.

Preface

At the time of writing, I have been supporting prospective university students with their university application for the past seven years and, in that time, I have amassed a wealth of experience and insight into the ingredients which go into composing an outstanding university Personal Statement. When I first began supporting individuals with their university application I found that the vast majority felt they received very little in the way of guidance – a situation which can only result in a below par Personal Statement and a significantly reduced chance of a successful application for those concerned. It was with this conviction to 'level the playing field' within the university application process that I made the decision to write this book.

According to UCAS, of the approximately 700,00 applicants to universities in the UK in 2010, around 490,000 were successful. To put it bluntly, around 70% of applicants were successful. To use an analogy, if you were in the Wild West and challenged to a game of Russian Roulette involving a pistol with one of its four bullet chambers loaded, would you consider a 70% chance of surviving good enough odds? Would you fancy your chances? It is precisely this situation which I am dedicated to addressing: removing the uncertainty from your university application.

Drawing upon my extensive experience of all aspects of applying to university, I embarked upon writing this guide in order to share my wisdom in planning, writing and improving a Personal Statement. This guide represents a comprehensive 'one-stop-shop' for all those intending to apply to a UK university via the Universities and College Admissions Service (UCAS), and who therefore must write a Personal Statement. In this guide I cover the entire university application process: from the initial decision to study at university to the final careful edit of your completed Personal Statement, along with everything in between.

Preface

The advice, suggestions, recommendations and tips included in this guide apply to many degree subjects, all types of student, including school leavers, mature and overseas students, as well as parents and teachers.

Please note that the examples contained within this book are for guidance purposes only and must not be used as part of your application. BPP Learning Media does not agree with plagiarised applications and fully supports the crackdown on plagiarism mounted by UCAS, through the use of electronic systems to counter applicants merely cutting and pasting examples into their own application.

I hope that you find this guide both informative and helpful and would like to wish you the best of luck with your university application.

Chapter 1

Applying to a Dental School in the United Kingdom: The process

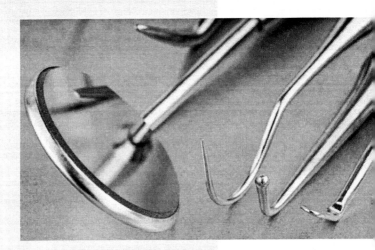

Applying to a Dental School in the United Kingdom: The process

In 2005 there were over 22,000 applications to study Medicine and Dentistry in the United Kingdom. Across the country, there are on average around five applications for each Dental School place on offer.

There are three steps in this application process:

- Sitting the appropriate entrance examination where applicable (some universities require Dentistry applicants to sit the UKCAT; examinations take place between June and October in the year before successful candidates begin their studies).
- Submitting a university application which includes the Personal Statement (mid-October deadline).
- Attending a selection interview when applicable (interviews take place between October and the following June depending upon the Dental School).

Dental School entrance examinations

An increasing number of Dental Schools require candidates to sit the United Kingdom Clinical Aptitude Test (UKCAT) before submitting their application. It is therefore important to determine as soon as possible whether or not the Dental Schools to which you intend to apply require you to sit this entrance examination. The UKCAT is based upon an aptitude format assessing a number of different criteria. The aim of this test is to aid the application process by ensuring that appropriate attitude, mental competence and professional qualities are specifically considered.

UKCAT

The UKCAT aptitude test was formally adopted in 2006 by a consortium of Medical and Dental Schools in the UK. The test is designed to assist admissions tutors select candidates who possess the desired mental abilities, approaches and attributes of successful dental students and practising dentists.

The test sets out to examine the following five qualities:

- Verbal reasoning
- Quantitative reasoning
- Abstract reasoning
- Decision analysis
- Non-cognitive analysis

Registration for the exam must be made directly through the UCKAT website. For more information visit:

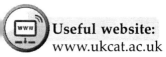 **Useful website:**
www.ukcat.ac.uk

The UCAS application

As the competition for Dental School places continues to increase, the need for a clear, engaging and well-structured university application is paramount. The Universities and Colleges Admission Service (UCAS) mediate applications made to universities in the United Kingdom through an online system (for more information visit www.ucas.com). If you are at school or college, the application process will be co-ordinated by the head of post-16 education and you will be provided with login details and instructions on how to proceed. If you are applying as a graduate or mature student not currently in full time education, you can register with UCAS directly in order to submit your application.

You cannot apply directly to a UK Dental School to study Dentistry. All applications must be made via UCAS using the somewhat daunting 'UCAS application form' which is now in electronic format. Although the paper-based 'UCAS form' is not commonly used now for applications to Dental School, the electronic application process still requires all of the information that would have been previously submitted. Accordingly, the electronic UCAS form requires you to enter your personal details, your course choices, your predicted or actual grades, your reference and your Personal Statement.

Dental School admissions tutors use the UCAS Personal Statement, as well as your A level or Higher grades and UKCAT results, when choosing which candidates to select to interview; it is crucial that this aspect of your application is of the highest quality. It is also important to note that when a candidate fails to achieve their target grades, the first thing an admissions tutor will look at when deciding whether to accept the applicant is their Personal Statement and their performance at any selection interview.

At present, the Dental School Personal Statement must be completed within 4,000 characters. It is also important to note that when entering the Personal Statement onto the UCAS system, any formatting – such as underlining, italics or bolding – will be lost.

So, **your** UCAS Personal Statement is **your** key opportunity to convince Dental School admissions tutors that **you** are an exceptional candidate and that they should offer **you** a place at their Dental School over other applicants.

It is vital that you make your comments clearly and compellingly, so that the admissions tutors become really keen to meet you and find out more about the special, unique person that you are!

Applying to study different subjects

Currently, candidates applying to study Dentistry are restricted to applying to four Dental Schools in a calendar year, whereas applicants for degree subjects other than Dentistry and Medicine are invited to apply to five universities. Accordingly, applicants to study Dentistry are also able to apply for one other non-clinical course, such as Pharmacy or Biomedical Sciences. However it is important to remember that within each candidate's application, only one Personal Statement can be submitted.

It is the advice of the authors, based upon their practical experience, that candidates seeking to study Dentistry should write their Personal Statement wholly with the aim of gaining acceptance to study Dentistry. Any attempt to incorporate other course choices would be inadvisable; such an approach would almost certainly reduce the strength of the Personal Statement.

Key points

Make sure that you first make contact with UCAS, the UKCAT examination website, and the Dental Schools themselves in order to find out *exactly* what you need to do when applying to study Dentistry.

Attending university Open Days is especially valuable; you have the chance then to ask questions directly.

Chapter 2

What kind of students do Dental Schools want?

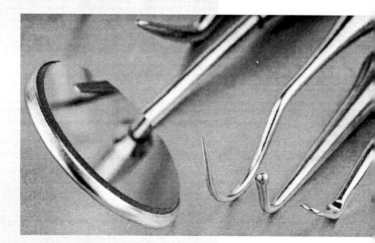

What kind of students do Dental Schools want?

Through our experience supporting individuals in their applications to study Dentistry, we have formed a solid understanding of the guiding principles used by Dental Schools in the selection and admission of students.

These are:

1. **Selection for Dental School implies selection for the dental profession**
   A degree in Dentistry confirms academic achievement and in normal circumstances entitles the new graduate to be provisionally registered by the General Dental Council.
2. The selection process attempts to identify the core academic and non-academic qualities of a dentist:
   - **Honesty, integrity** and an ability to **recognise one's own limitations** and those of others, are central to the practice of dentistry.
   - Other key attributes include having **good communication** and **listening skills,** an ability **to make decisions under pressure**, and to **remain calm and cope with stress.**
   - Dentists must have an understanding of **teamwork** and respect for the contributions of others. Desirable characteristics include **curiosity, creativity, initiative, flexibility** and **leadership.**
3. A high level of academic attainment will be expected. **Understanding science is core to the understanding of dentistry**, but Dental Schools generally encourage diversity in subjects studied by candidates.
4. The practice of dentistry requires the highest standards of **professional** and **personal conduct**. Put simply, some students will not be suited to a career in dentistry and it

is in the interests of the student and the public that they should not be admitted to Dental School.

5. The practice of dentistry requires the highest standards of **professional competence**. However, a history of serious ill health or disability will not jeopardise a career in dentistry unless the condition impinges upon professional fitness to practise.

6. Candidates should demonstrate some understanding of what a career in dentistry involves and their suitability for a caring profession. Dental Schools expect candidates to have had some relevant experience in oral health or related areas. Indeed, some Dental Schools stipulate a defined minimum period of relevant work experience.

7. The **primary duty of care is to patients.** All applicants to Dental Schools will be expected to understand the importance of this principle.

8. Failure to declare information that has a material influence on a student's fitness to practise may lead to termination of their dental course.

Clearly, it is important that you consult the websites of the Dental Schools to which you intend to apply in order to learn of any specific requirements they are seeking.

University education is also expensive. For every dental student who drops out, there are financial implications to the university.

So, one of the most important questions to be considered by a Dental School is: will the student complete the course?

Finally, Dental Schools are also looking for students who will contribute to the broad spectrum of university life. Those who do so are so much more likely to gain a wider experience of working and communicating with people from different backgrounds.

The admissions tutor's perspective

In deciding who will and who will not to be invited to study Dentistry at their university, Dental Schools look to the views of their admissions tutors, the people who read the application submissions and who conduct the interviews.

And when reading hundreds of Personal Statements, so often the key considerations of the tutors are:

'Does this candidate have a sense of what they are going to get into by studying Dentistry, and indeed by studying Dentistry at this Dental School?'

'Can I see this individual becoming a good practicing dentist in a few years from now?'

Whilst it is likely that admissions tutors will be looking to see if you possess the personal qualities so often associated with dentists – qualities such as kindness, compassion, empathy, and curiosity – they are perhaps even more determined to see if you are always reliable, and that you can handle the physical, mental and emotional strains you will experience, firstly as a dental student and then as a professional practitioner.

Key points

Selection for Dental School implies selection for the dental profession.

Dental Schools want candidates with more than academic ability. They want to train the dentists of tomorrow.

Chapter 3

The essential contents of the Personal Statement

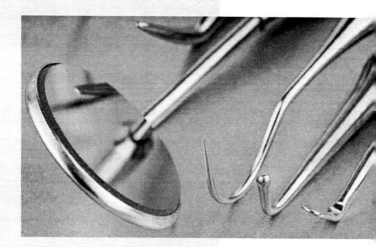

The essential contents of the Personal Statement

Your Personal Statement is your opportunity to describe in words:

- The reasons why you are so keen to study Dentistry, and at the universities to which you are submitting your applications.
- That even in advance of taking up your dental studies, you have already made a real commitment to this course of action by gaining relevant experience.
- That you have a good idea of, and are equipped to handle, the expectations, responsibilities, pressures and duties attached to the practice of dentistry.
- That you are special, and possess attributes which will see you through your dental course and towards establishing your professional career.

Let us take each of these themes above and look at them carefully.

What is Dentistry?

'Dentistry is a professional clinical discipline concerned with prevention, detection, management and treatment of oral and dental diseases and maintenance of oral and dental health, in individuals and in society. It is based on sound scientific and technical principles with the clinical aspects of dentistry underpinned by knowledge and understanding of the biological and clinical medical sciences. Graduates from dental schools are required to demonstrate a thorough understanding of the importance of ethical practice and professionalism, high levels of ability in communication skills and competence in the clinical and technical aspects of dentistry.'

UCAS website June 2010

Every would-be dental student has their own story as to how and why they came to make that academic and career choice. In your Personal Statement, it is vital that you explain **your** own journey in **your** own **unique** way. But you must present your story with real **conviction**.

During our years of experience we have been in contact with many successful dental practitioners, all with their own unique reasons for entering the profession. Their accounts are incredibly illuminating and worth considering when preparing your Personal Statement.

Here are some of their comments:

> *'As is hopefully true for all dentists, I am inspired by the opportunity to spend my professional lifetime trying to improve the health and welfare of humanity. I always believed that no higher calling existed than to help individual patients.'*

> *'I find it hard to look back and capture what initially inspired me to take up dentistry, but I think that my aspirations are still the same. Dentistry is a "way of life" and combines that rather nebulous feeling of wanting to help and care with the more exact principles of science and logical thought. After all these years as a dentist, I still want to get out of bed and go to work in the mornings.'*

> *'Dentists are among the top list of professionals that the public thinks are worthy of "respect" and also are "most likely to tell the truth", and this makes me feel privileged to be a dentist.'*

> *'There is no place for arrogance or self-satisfaction. I still relish a challenge that calls on all my faculties and training. I have been fortunate to treat people from different ethnic groups with different cultures, beliefs and diseases. This has been a humbling experience but also educational and fascinating.'*

'Dentistry offers a huge variety of choices – clinical work, research, teaching, training and management – to name but a few. Dentistry is currently undergoing many changes. The dental curriculum has changed almost beyond recognition since I was a student. More emphasis is placed on communication and clinical skills. The greatest joy is that simple "thank you" as the patient walks out of the door. Isn't it great?'

'Dentistry is based on altruism, science, and human interest. Like most dental students, this is what attracted me and it still does. The aspirations are of excellent care, progress, and change. I find the continuing movement, and certainty that we will know more, inspirational and energising. Dentistry is remarkable in its clinical and scientific breadth and its fusion with other disciplines and interests. Much of dentistry grows from basic biology, but dental research and practice is also linked to physics, chemistry, statistics, population science, sociology and politics.'

'Whatever interests and personality you have, there is probably an aspect of dentistry to suit you. The diversity can be confusing for a student and young dentist thinking about a career. When I qualified I did not know what would be the best path to choose.'

'Teaching and training are essential components of dentistry. Brilliant lectures and articles and new discoveries and ideas are great rejuvenators. The constant development of new approaches is engrossing.'

Clearly, these accounts are written with the wisdom which comes after many years of dental experience. But the statements really do deserve careful consideration; they were written by dentists, to be read, very largely, by other dentists.

For example, look at the way these authors describe their enthusiasm for dentistry: in particular, note the use of words such as *'inspired'*, *'aspirations'*, *'relish'*, *'energising'*, *'engrossing'*.

Look also at their references to the challenges and uncertainties which accompany dental studies. For example, *'The diversity can be confusing for a student'* and *'When I qualified I did not know what would be the best path to choose'*.

When writing your own Personal Statement, you must write in your own style. However, you can be sure that admissions tutors are looking to see evidence of **enthusiasm** and careful **reflection** in your comments.

Why Dentistry at this university?

Before you begin to write your Personal Statement you need to decide the Dental Schools to which you wish to apply. It is important that you consult a careers advisor and visit the Dental Schools yourself before making your final decision. This is a decision not to be taken lightly given the fact that you will be dedicating the next several years to studying there.

There are many factors to take into account when considering your choice, including:

- Would you prefer to study at a campus or city-based Dental School?
- Do you feel comfortable in the locality in which the Dental School is set?
- Are you happy with the educational approaches taken by the Dental Schools under consideration? These do vary. For example, some courses concentrate on Problem-Based Learning, a style of teaching which is based on the consideration of case studies, or scenarios, and the students presenting their findings in the context of achieving defined educational objectives.
- When would you start interacting with patients?
- What extracurricular activities are available?
- Do you want to study close to your family home, or not?

Each Dental School has a slightly different selection process so it is important that you also visit their website in order to obtain the necessary details.

Your commitment to dental studies and a dental career

Consider the situation in which a Premier League football club is deliberating whether or not to offer a teenage boy, with aspirations to be a professional footballer, a position within the club's youth academy. You can be sure that in addition to their consideration of his football ability, the club's coaches will also be looking to see signs of a real commitment to a future career in the sport as demonstrated by, for example, his approach to diet, and his attitude to drinking and smoking. In short, the club will be keen to see evidence of personal investment in this career move. What is he keen to do; what is he prepared to give up?

The same applies in the consideration of Dental School applications. The admissions tutors will be keen to find out how you spend your time outside the formal school curriculum.

For example, they may look to see if your Personal Statement contains evidence that:

- You try to keep abreast of dental developments as they are reported in leading dental journals, such as *The BDJ*, and the national newspapers, or
- You have gained knowledge of the dental profession through relevant work experience.

Understanding the expectations, responsibilities and duties attached to the practice of dentistry

The most authoritative description of the responsibilities and duties of dentists working in the United Kingdom is that issued by the General Dental Council (GDC), the body with which all dental practitioners in the UK must become registered.

Presented below are the six defining principles of practice laid out by the GDC in 'Standards for Dental Professionals'. **It is imperative that all applicants to Dental School gain a full understanding of the GDC's requirements.**

The duties of a dentist registered with the General Dental Council

As a registered member of the GDC, you are responsible for:

1. **Putting patients' interests first and acting to protect them:**
    *   *Adopt patient priority as your guiding principle; never promote your own, or the interests of your business, over those of the public.*
    *   *Respect the patients' right to seek alternative consultation, to decline treatment, or to lodge a complaint; ensure appropriate procedures are followed under these circumstances.*
    *   *Act immediately if you believe the health, behaviour or performance of you or a colleague may be putting the patient at risk.*

2. **Respecting patients' dignity and choices:**
    *   *Adopt a polite and respectful approach toward patient care; respect the rights of each individual and do not discriminate.*
    *   *Effectively communicate with patients to ensure they are able to make fully informed decisions; never take action without full consent from the patient.*

- Actively engage with patients to promote responsibility for oral healthcare.

3. **Protecting the confidentiality of patients' information:**
   - Only use patient information for the purpose for which it was given and adopt responsibility for preventing any unauthorised access.
   - On occasion, it may be acceptable to share confidential information without consent if it is in the interest of the public, or indeed, the patient. In these exceptional circumstances, seek guidance from the GDC before taking action.

4. **Co-operating with other members of the dental team and other healthcare colleagues in the interest of patients:**
   - Work effectively as part of a team, sharing knowledge and skills where necessary, to ensure the best possible standards of patient care.
   - Treat all colleagues with respect; do not discriminate.

5. **Maintaining your professional knowledge and competence:**
   - Recognise that you are responsible for continued professional development through lifelong learning; continually assess and update your knowledge and performance.
   - Work within the confines of your skills and follow up to date guidelines for best practice in your relevant field.
   - Understand and adhere to relevant regulations affecting both your work and your working environment.

6. **Being trustworthy:**
   - Maintain the trust of the public, your patients and your colleagues through open, honest and professional behaviour.
   - Recognise that you are responsible for upholding confidence, not only in yourself as a dental practitioner, but in the dental profession as a whole.

Show them you are special

When considering the Personal Statements of applicants to Dental Schools, the admissions tutors will also be asking themselves:

- *Has this applicant really thought things through?*
- *Do we want to meet this candidate at interview?*
- *Do we see them enjoying and completing their studies, well on their way to becoming a good dentist?*
- *Will it be good for the university to have this candidate around?*

Your Personal Statement is your opportunity to influence the tutors towards saying 'Yes' in response to each of these questions as they apply to you!

So, it is important that you write in a way that depicts the enthusiasm, keenness – and indeed, **passion** – you have for your chosen academic choice.

Phrases such as 'I am *quite* interested in studying Dentistry' or 'I really *think* that Dentistry is the right course for me' are to be avoided; they are so unconvincing! And if you have received special commendations or prizes, write about them in a way that shows how they reinforce your decision to study Dentistry.

For example, if you became Head Pupil at your school, this clearly shows the strength of the teachers' regard for your leadership qualities, and your ability to act as a role model for other pupils. So, elaborate upon those themes. Equally, if you worked effectively as part of a team raising money for your school's charity, you could describe how this experience improved your teamwork and communication skills.

It is vitally important when referring to your experiences in your Personal Statement to clearly state how these have developed in you the qualities that are required of a dental student and future dentist.

However, before you submit your final statement, you would also do well to talk about your 'special' qualities with your referee. Some comments are simply more effectively made by another person and it is important that your reference fully supports your application to Dental School.

Key point

It is vital that you use your Personal Statement to convince the admissions tutors that you have really considered the implications of studying Dentistry **and** that you know that it is right for you.

Chapter 4

Dental School applications: The myths

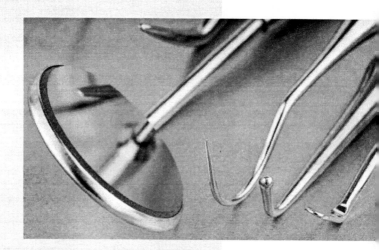

Dental School applications: The myths

During our experience in supporting students in their applications to Dental Schools, we have come across many misunderstandings. Here are some which arise time after time:

1. **Dental Schools are keen to meet students whose key motivation for wishing to become a dentist is due to a parent being a dentist.**

   No. Clearly, the fact that one of your parents is a dentist may very significantly account for your keen interest in studying Dentistry. However, this is simply not sufficient justification for your decision to embark upon a dental career. Admissions tutors will be looking to see how you have carefully considered your career options, and how you have confirmed your final choice by gaining appropriate experience.

2. **It is easier to get into Dental School if your parent is a dentist.**

   This is not true. Again, if your parent is a dentist it is certainly easier to gain an insight into the world of dentistry. However, Dental Schools are interested in each individual applicant and in the steps they have undertaken to confirm that they have the right qualities for a future dental career.

3. **Dental Schools are much more likely to accept students from private schools.**

   This simply is not true – Dental Schools look to offer places to the best candidates regardless of whether they attended a private or state school. Your suitability for gaining an interview and subsequent place will be determined by the quality of your university application, including particularly the effort that you have placed in preparing your Personal Statement. Remember, together with your predicted grades, it is predominantly the strength of your

Personal Statement and your reference that will determine whether you are invited to attend an interview or not.

4. **I am the first person to ever apply to Dental School from my school, therefore I don't stand a chance of being accepted.**

This is not true and a common misconception. Simply because you may be the first person from your school or college to apply to study Dentistry does not mean that your chances are reduced. Successful candidates are those who have invested time and effort in preparing their applications, and who have ensured that their referees became aware of their keen intentions to study Dentistry.

5. **I must achieve all A grades in my GCSEs and my A levels to get into Dental School.**

This is not necessarily true and depends on the particular Dental School and its entry requirements. It is therefore important that you carefully study the admissions criteria of the Dental Schools to which you intend to apply.

6. **Scoring well in my examinations is the only thing I need to do to get into Dental School.**

Not true at all. Yes, successful applicants to Dental Schools will obtain excellent academic results; however, it is vital that they also demonstrate that they have the qualities required of a good dentist. Think back to your own experiences when you were treated by a dentist: what special qualities made them stand out? Some of these include:

- Having a real desire to help people.
- Being able to communicate clearly.
- Understanding the importance of effective team working and leadership skills.
- Being empathic and honest.
- Recognising the importance of adopting a conscientious and highly motivated approach.

7. **When describing your work experience you should not refer to non-dental experience.**

   It is important to refer to your dental and your non-dental experiences to demonstrate how these have helped to equip you in your forthcoming studies, and beyond. For example, someone describing that they had led a mountaineering expedition would clearly demonstrate their strong leadership and team working skills.

8. **My Personal Statement must be exactly 4,000 characters or I will be penalised.**

   Obviously, the more relevant information you include within the allowed space then the more fully you will be able to tell the admissions tutors about yourself and why you should be offered a place at their Dental School. However, it really is about quality not quantity, so do not attempt to pad out your Personal Statement with irrelevant facts that do not add any value to your application or, worse still, weaken it.

9. **The sooner I submit my Personal Statement before the deadline the better my chances of success.**

   This is another common misconception. The only real advantage of submitting your Dental School application as early as possible is that it will reduce your stress levels and enable you to concentrate on your studies. Despite what is commonly perceived, submitting your application earlier rather than later will not mean that you stand a better chance of your application progressing simply because it is at the top of the admission tutor's pile!

10. **If I select one other course choice in addition to Dentistry I will reduce my chances.**

    Admissions tutors will not think that you are less committed to studying Dentistry if you list one other course in addition to the four Dental School applications you have submitted. Indeed, unless the courses you have selected are at the same university, the Data Protection Act precludes admissions tutors the ability to identify your other applications.

However, it is important that your Personal Statement is 100 per cent tailored to your application to study Dentistry and does not contain reference to other non-dental courses.

Key point

Your Personal Statement is your opportunity to justify to the admissions tutors why **you**, as a **unique individual**, should be accepted to Dental School in the first step of a dental career.

Chapter 5

Preparing your Personal Statement

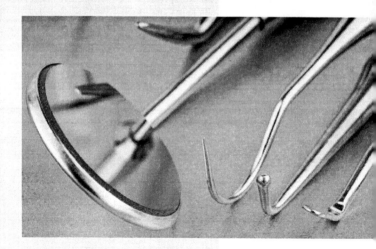

Chapter 5

Preparing your Personal Statement

Check the key questions

The first step in preparing your Personal Statement is to take a good look at yourself – your personality, your strengths and your achievements. Then take a blank piece of paper and write down where you stand with regard to the key questions set out below. It is almost certain that you will not be able to touch upon each and every topic covered by these questions in your final Personal Statement. However, it will be helpful for you to consider each question; you can then decide which areas you are keen to include and which ones you are content to discard.

You might also find it valuable to have to hand the following when considering the key questions below:

- The list of 'Duties of a dentist registered with the General Dental Council' (page 17).
- The guiding principles adopted in the selection and admission of students to Dental Schools (page 8).
- The quotations from dental professionals (pages 13–14).

But please note: it is extremely important that when it comes to writing your Personal Statement, you create your own expressions and phrases. Your Personal Statement has to be written uniquely in your style – about you!

Key questions

- When and why did you begin to be interested in dentistry?
- Why do you want to study Dentistry? Are you sure you want to be a dentist? Why do you want to be a dentist rather than, for example, a dental nurse, or a doctor? Or a lawyer?

28

- Why are you so keen to study Dentistry at this particular university?
- What kind of person are you? Which aspects of your personality equip you well for dental studies and a career in dentistry?
- What are your strengths and weaknesses? What are your strengths and weaknesses according to others, such as your parents, your friends, your teachers? What special talents do you have which could be of real value within a dental career?
- What work experience have you had which has given you a special insight into life as a dental student or as a dentist?
- What else have you done, or has happened to you, which has provided excellent learning experiences or drawn upon your special personal qualities, such as compassion, tenacity, empathy?
- What awards or prizes (academic and non-academic) have you received? What do these tell people about you?
- What are your keen interests outside academic studies?
- What do you see yourself doing in five or ten years' time?

Drafting a structure

When complete, an effective Personal Statement will comprise **three key sections**: your 'introduction', a 'conclusion', and between these two sections will lie those paragraphs comprising the 'main body' of the Personal Statement.

It is helpful to sketch onto a piece of blank paper three boxes; one labelled 'Introduction', one labelled 'Conclusion' and, lying between those two boxes, one labelled 'Main body'.

Now start mapping some draft comments to each of the three sections.

The introduction

The aim of the introduction is to catch the attention of the reader, namely the admissions tutor. So, try to compose a statement which really grabs the reader's attention and enables you to stand out from the crowd!

The main body of the Personal Statement

The main body of your Personal Statement is the section in which you build upon your introduction and describe:

- Why you have decided to study Dentistry.
- The steps you have taken in making a real commitment to study Dentistry.
- How you have a real sense of what dental studies and a subsequent dental career entail.
- Aspects of yourself which especially equip you for this course of action.

It is in this section that you will refer to:

- Your work experience, and the relevant insights it has given you towards confirming that studying Dentistry is right for you.
- The steps you have taken in furthering your interest in dentistry and dental matters.
- The topics which you look forward to studying most.
- Your experience of teamwork, leadership and responsibility, reliability and tenacity.
- Your thoughts upon what direction your dental career might take, always recognising that this might change in the light of experience at Dental School.

The conclusion

It is vitally important to draw your Personal Statement to a close, and reaffirm that you are someone who will flourish academically and socially at Dental School, and that you are well equipped to handle the stresses and strains associated with dental studies. The 'conclusion' paragraph is not the time to introduce any new themes. However, not to present a concise, summary comment would be a real error of judgement.

Writing and improving your Personal Statement

In formulating the contents of each of the key sections (introduction; main body; conclusion) of your Personal Statement, it is important that you focus upon the following questions:

- Do each of your sections, **especially the introduction,** and your Personal Statement as a whole have **real impact upon the reader?**
- Is the punctuation correct?
- Is the flow of your language appealing, non-repetitive and easy to follow?
- Is there a logical and coherent balance to the Personal Statement?
- Are all your statements absolutely honest and accurate? Remember! Anything you refer to in your Personal Statement may be the subject of questions at any subsequent interviews. Admissions tutors are very skilled at identifying situations where candidates have made exaggerated claims!
- Will the reader conclude that you are indeed 'special'? Is it truly about you?

And finally:

- **Have you concentrated on justifying and substantiating your comments?**

The admissions tutors will consider everything that you include in your Personal Statement to help them decide whether or not to offer you the opportunity to study Dentistry at their university. It is not enough to write, for example: *'I want to study Dentistry*

because Biology is my strongest subject, academically.' To excel in a specific academic subject is simply not sufficient justification for seeking to make a career within dentistry and all that it entails.

Look again at this statement from the quotations presented earlier in Chapter 3:

> *'I find it hard to look back and capture what initially inspired me to take up dentistry, but I think that my aspirations are still the same. Dentistry is a "way of life" and combines that rather nebulous feeling of wanting to help and care with the more exact principles of science and logical thought.'*

This writer provides clear evidence that it was the combination of their joy in scientific intellectual stimulation and the opportunity to reach out and support others that inspired them to study Dentistry and develop a dental career.

You must maintain your own focus upon justifying and substantiating your comments throughout your entire Personal Statement.

Key points

You need time to write your Personal Statement, do not rush.

Prepare a first **draft**, containing an introduction, a main body and a conclusion.

Chapter 6

From 'Draft' to 'Refined': enhancing your Personal Statement

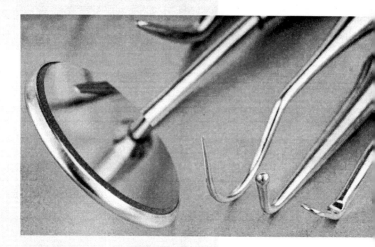

From 'Draft' to 'Refined': enhancing your Personal Statement

One way in which we can illustrate the importance of focusing upon the key principles which govern the preparation of an effective, compelling Personal Statement is to consider a fictitious example, initially in its first 'draft' form, and then looking at it after some refinement. The critique which follows should not be interpreted as 'definitive', or 'state of the art'. And certainly, there is no such thing as the perfect Personal Statement. However, we hope that by using this scenario – moving from a 'draft' to a 'refined' version – we can bring the whole process to life!

Fictitious Personal Statement: 'Draft' version

I am applying for this course because I am very interested in becoming a dentist. I have been interested in this career since I was young. I became fascinated in the subject when I started having orthodontic treatment when I was eight and at school I am very interested in human biology. I have been inspired by an uncle who is a dentist and for the last three years I have helped to care for my elderly grandmother. This opportunity has helped me to see the satisfaction gained from working within the caring professions.

My AS levels are very relevant to this course and I have specifically chosen to continue Chemistry, Biology and Maths to A2 level so that I can apply to dentistry. I also enjoy reading science magazines and books by writers such as Stephen Hawking. In order to understand the subject more clearly I have been to a careers fair featuring a talk about careers in dentistry. This has further inspired me towards dentistry as my profession of choice. I have also arranged to undergo some work experience at Hope Medical Practice in Wakefield and at Gerald Barrer Associates, a much larger practice in Dewsbury. This gave me an insight into how a dental practice is run. During my placement I worked in various areas including working within the

reception area, answering the phone, making appointments, using the computer system and observing dental treatments. Once a month for the last three years I have helped to look after my grandmother who has Alzheimer's disease by helping her to eat, wash and dress. A dentist needs to have strong empathy for his patients, especially when they are nervous, therefore looking after my grandmother has helped me to understand how to do this.

In my free time I enjoy voluntary work, leisure activities and part time work. At the moment I have just started a new job as a part time care assistant at a nursing home. I am enjoying caring for the patients and talking to them to help them feel at ease. My colleagues are of various different ages and backgrounds and this has helped me to develop my confidence and communication skills. As well as my job I like to participate in my school's enrichment programme and on the Duke of Edinburgh Bronze Award. The music enrichment classes have enabled me to learn to play the keyboards and I enjoy practising this at home. I am currently working towards my Duke of Edinburgh Bronze Award and so far I have completed the community and the expedition parts of this award. For my community work I helped at an Oxfam shop which has given me experience of customer service and using the till. For the expedition I took part in a hiking trip to Bavaria, during which we completed 21 miles over two days. Both of these helped me experience different types of team work. I also enjoy attending football matches in my free time.

Character count: 2,827

Fictitious Personal Statement: 'Refined' version

A career in Dentistry appeals to me as it will allow me to develop both my fascination for human biology and my enjoyment of helping others. Discussions with dentists have given me a realistic appreciation of both the challenges and rewards of this profession and my work experience has helped me to confirm my commitment to a role requiring self-motivation, interpersonal skills and great attention to detail.

At A level I have found the hands-on aspects of the Sciences particularly engaging, utilising both my manual dexterity and my logical approach to problem solving. In Physics I have enjoyed learning about the ways in which the properties and functions of different materials are used to address real life issues. Researching oral hygiene for my Biology coursework allowed me to pursue my interest in dental physiology as well as developing my experience of analysing large quantities of qualitative and quantitative information. Self-directed reading of books such as those by Stephen Hawking and James Gleick has significantly broadened my scientific knowledge. As a subscriber to New Scientist and Nature magazines I keep myself informed on developments within scientific research; recently I have followed reports on new technologies such as the 'plasma needle' with interest as these will have a great impact on dental surgery in the future. I find it fascinating to read about the ways in which surgery has changed over the last two centuries and to consider what developments there will be during my own career. I am looking forward to the opportunity to discuss issues such as these at university and especially to studying the theory and techniques of oral surgery.

A two week work experience placement at a general dental practice has given me an insight into the day to day duties and responsibilities of a dentist, from cleaning teeth and filling cavities to diagnosing gum disease and giving advice on oral hygiene. I was surprised by the level of interaction and teamwork with other members of staff and I enjoyed learning about how dentistry fits in with the rest of the NHS. Several patients, for example, were referred to their GPs, and another had been receiving reconstructive maxillofacial treatment from a team made up of dentists, surgeons and nurses. A further week at a larger practice allowed me to observe specialists in several areas and I made the most of this opportunity to learn about the different career paths available. During both of these placements I helped to reassure the patients, enhancing my oral communication skills. I found working with the more nervous patients especially rewarding as I was able to make a real difference to their experience. In addition, assisting the receptionist allowed me to utilise my organisational skills. A careers talk on dentistry deepened my understanding of the training and career structures and helped to confirm my interest in this profession. My

job as a care assistant has furthered my healthcare experience and I have learnt about ethical issues such as confidentiality and patient consent. My interpersonal skills have also been enhanced through my role as a part time carer for my elderly grandmother, which requires me to provide regular personal care.

Learning to play the keyboard has provided me with an interesting creative outlet and composing pieces in several parts requires co-ordination and an eye for detail. At present I am also working towards my Bronze Duke of Edinburgh Award; volunteering at a charity shop has allowed me to contribute to my community and through completing a two day expedition I have enhanced my skills in both teamwork and leadership.

In conclusion, I consider myself a hardworking and well-rounded student and I look forward to making full use of the opportunities available to me at university.

Character count: 3,827

Improving your Personal Statement

The following analysis aims to help you to create an engaging Personal Statement by looking at ways the 'draft' statement was refined. By considering the 'draft' and 'refined' paragraphs side by side, important principles can be highlighted.

Paragraph one: Draft

'I am applying for this course because I am very interested in becoming a dentist. I have been interested in this career since I was young. I became fascinated in the subject when I started having orthodontic treatment when I was eight and at school I am very interested in human biology. I have been inspired by an uncle who is a dentist and for the last three years I have helped to care for my elderly grandmother. This opportunity has helped me to see the satisfaction gained from working within the caring professions.'

Paragraph one: Refined

'A career in Dentistry appeals to me as it will allow me to develop both my fascination for human biology and my enjoyment of helping others. Discussions with dentists have given me a realistic appreciation of both the challenges and rewards of this profession and my work experience has helped me to confirm my commitment to a role requiring self-motivation, interpersonal skills and great attention to detail.'

Paragraph one: Draft

The opening sentences here are repetitive and unoriginal. It is unlikely that anyone will apply for Dentistry unless they intend to become a dentist, so there is no need to waste words by pointing this out. You should also beware of claiming to have 'always' wanted to be a dentist or saying that it has been your childhood ambition. The admissions panel read hundreds of opening sentences like this and it does not give them any information about how you stand out from the other applicants. Even if dentistry really is what you have always wanted to do, it can seem naïve to state this as your main reason for applying – as a young child you would not have had a good understanding of what this career involves. Instead, you should demonstrate to the admissions panel that your decision to apply for Dentistry is based on well-considered and logical reasons rather than childhood ambitions.

Remember to assign a capital letter to the title of the degree course, i.e. Dentistry not dentistry, and avoid beginning sentences with 'I' as this sounds unsophisticated and is repetitive to read. You want your admissions tutor to find reading your Personal Statement enjoyable and interesting!

Beware of mentioning relatives or friends who are already studying or practicing as dentists unless you can justify how this has helped you to make your decision. For example, you may have learned from them about the training structure of dentistry or about the different specialties available.

Paragraph one: Refined

The opening paragraph now begins with a concise and logical summary of the applicant's reasons for applying. This provides a more engaging start and sets a confident, active tone to the paragraph. The applicant then demonstrates that they have worked hard to become well-informed about the realities of a career in dentistry and shows that they have not made their decision lightly. Remember that it is more effective to demonstrate that you are well-informed by mentioning some of the qualities a dentist needs (e.g. self-motivation, interpersonal skills) than to simply state *'I am well-informed about what Dentistry involves'*. You should aim to *show* the admissions tutors that you have the required qualities rather than *tell* them that you do. The more varied sentence structure keeps the reader engaged and demonstrates that the applicant is capable of a more mature writing style.

Paragraph two: Draft

'My AS levels are very relevant to this course and I have specifically chosen to continue Chemistry, Biology and Maths to A2 level so that I can apply to dentistry. I also enjoy reading science magazines and books by writers such as Stephen Hawking. In order to understand the subject more clearly I have been to a careers fair featuring a talk about careers in dentistry. This has further inspired me towards dentistry as my profession of choice.'

Paragraph two: Refined

'*At A level I have found the hands-on aspects of the Sciences particularly engaging, utilising both my manual dexterity and my logical approach to problem solving. In Physics I have enjoyed learning about the ways in which the properties and functions of different materials are used to address real life issues. Researching oral hygiene for my Biology coursework allowed me to pursue my interest in dental physiology as well as developing my experience of analysing large quantities of qualitative and quantitative information. Self-directed reading of books such as those by Stephen Hawking and James Gleick has significantly broadened my scientific knowledge. As a subscriber to New Scientist and Nature magazines I keep myself informed on developments within scientific research; recently I have followed reports on new technologies such as the 'plasma needle' with interest as these will have a great impact on dental surgery in the future. I find it fascinating to read about the ways in which surgery has changed over the last two centuries and to consider what developments there will be during my own career. I am looking forward to the opportunity to discuss issues such as these at university and especially to studying the theory and techniques of oral surgery.*'

Paragraph two: Draft

This paragraph needlessly repeats information about AS and A2 subjects which is given elsewhere on the UCAS form. Remember that repeating information in this way not only wastes words but also indicates to the admissions tutor that you have not put much thought into writing your statement. Again it is important to consider what will make you stand out from the crowd of applicants; remember that most of your fellow applicants will have studied similar subjects and achieved similar grades. There is no need, therefore, to emphasise that you have chosen Science A levels.

Although it is useful to mention extra-curricular reading, there is no merit in simply listing authors or titles – anyone can copy out a list of impressive sounding names from a website. The applicant states that they like books about science, but this is not supported by any examples and there is no indication of what they have learnt from this. Instead, you need to demonstrate your enthusiasm for actually reading relevant books/magazines/newspapers by discussing what interests you about them.

The sentence referring to the applicant's attendance at a careers fair has been moved to paragraph three as it is more closely related to work experience than to academic work. Think carefully about the structure of your Personal Statement and try to keep related ideas together in one paragraph. This makes it easier to read and shows admissions tutors that you are well-organised and logical and that you have skills in written communication.

Paragraph two: Refined

This paragraph is your opportunity to demonstrate that you are academically engaged and that you enjoy the learning process. The admissions tutors want to see that you are committed to several years of rigorous study as well as to a later career as a dentist.

The applicant goes into much greater detail about why they have enjoyed their subjects. It is not necessary to list every single thing that you have enjoyed studying, but by highlighting one or two topics you have an opportunity to convey your enthusiasm for science and for learning in general. By mentioning the skills acquired in research and those gained in conducting experiments, the applicant shows self-awareness of the ways they have prepared themselves for university study. Mentioning current issues within clinical science which interest them shows not only that the applicant is reading outside school, but also what they are learning from this. As well as knowledge of topics related to dentistry, this can also be an opportunity to demonstrate that you have learnt wider academic skills such as conducting self-directed research and delivering presentations.

The paragraph concludes with a reference to the topics the student is particularly looking forward to studying at university. This provides a further opportunity to convey your enthusiasm for the subject and also shows that you have investigated and understood what your future degree will entail.

Paragraph three: Draft

'I have also arranged to undergo some work experience at Hope Medical Practice in Wakefield and at Gerald Barrer Associates, a much larger practice in Dewsbury. This gave me an insight into how a dental practice is run. During my placement I worked in various areas including working within the reception area, answering the phone, making appointments, using the computer system and observing dental treatments. Once a month for the last three years I have helped to look after my grandmother who has Alzheimer's disease by helping her to eat, wash and dress. A dentist needs to have strong empathy for his patients, especially when they are nervous, therefore looking after my grandmother has helped me to understand how to do this.'

Paragraph three: Refined

'A two week work experience placement at a general dental practice has given me an insight into the day to day duties and responsibilities of a dentist, from cleaning teeth and filling cavities to diagnosing gum disease and giving advice on oral hygiene. I was surprised by the level of interaction and teamwork with other members of staff and I enjoyed learning about how dentistry fits in with the rest of the NHS. Several patients, for example, were referred to their GPs, and another had been receiving reconstructive surgeons and nurses maxillofacial treatment from a team made up of dentists, . A further week at a larger practice allowed me to observe specialists in several areas and I made the most of this opportunity to learn about the different career paths available. During both of these placements I helped to reassure the patients, enhancing my oral

> *communication skills. I found working with the more nervous patients especially rewarding as I was able to make a real difference to their experience. In addition, assisting the receptionist allowed me to utilise my organisational skills. A careers talk on dentistry deepened my understanding of the training and career structures and helped to confirm my interest in this profession. My job as a care assistant has furthered my healthcare experience and I have learnt about ethical issues such as confidentiality and patient consent. My interpersonal skills have also been enhanced through my role as a part time carer for my elderly grandmother, which requires me to provide regular personal care.'*

Paragraph three: Draft

This paragraph is far too brief for what should be one of the main sections of your Personal Statement and does not give enough emphasis to dental work experience. There is no need to waste words by giving the name and location of the places you have worked at; these places will not be familiar to the admissions tutors anyway. By only mentioning dental observation at the end of a long list of clerical duties, the applicant has missed an opportunity to show what they have gained from the experience and how it has helped to inform their career choice. Relevant work experience and an awareness of how this has been beneficial for you is one of the key areas in which you can make your application stand out from the competition.

Paragraph three: Refined

This paragraph now forms a key part of the Personal Statement, showing the breadth of experience the applicant has and how it has helped them to decide on a career in dentistry. There are no unnecessary details, and the applicant discusses in depth what they learnt about dentistry. Mentioning specific experiences which surprised or particularly interested you is a good way of letting a little of your personality through and helps to prevent the paragraph becoming a list of achievements with no reflection. The applicant has clearly thought about what they gained from their work experiences, in terms of both practical skills, such as personal care, and wider issues such as confidentiality. The job as a carer is mentioned here, where it is most relevant.

Paragraph four: Draft

'In my free time I enjoy voluntary work, leisure activities and part time work. At the moment I have just started a new job as a part time care assistant at a nursing home. I am enjoying caring for the patients and talking to them to help them feel at ease. My colleagues are of various different ages and backgrounds and this has helped me to develop my confidence and communication skills. As well as my job I like to participate in my school's enrichment programme and on the Duke of Edinburgh Bronze Award. The music enrichment classes have enabled me to learn to play the keyboards and I enjoy practising this at home. I am currently working towards my Duke of Edinburgh Bronze Award and so far I have completed the community and the expedition parts of this award. For my community work I helped at an Oxfam shop which has given me experience of customer service and using the till. For the expedition I took part in a hiking trip to Bavaria, during which we completed 21 miles over two days. Both of these helped me experience different types of team work. I also enjoy attending football matches in my free time.'

Paragraph four: Refined

'Learning to play the keyboard has provided me with an interesting creative outlet and composing pieces in several parts requires co-ordination and an eye for detail. At present I am also working towards my Bronze Duke of Edinburgh Award; volunteering at a charity shop has allowed me to contribute to my community and through completing a two day expedition I have enhanced my skills in both teamwork and leadership.

Paragraph four: Draft

The paragraph in which you discuss extra-curricular interests should not dominate your Personal Statement and it should not read as a list of hobbies. This applicant has wasted a lot of words by repeating themselves; brainstorm your ideas first and then decide how you can make your point in a concise and simple way. The section on working at a care home, which is relevant healthcare work experience, should not be buried within a paragraph about leisure activities.

If you do have significant achievements, such as playing sport or music at a very high level, then you should highlight these here. However, the most important thing is to show that you understand how your hobbies, at whatever level of achievement, have developed you as a person. It is far better to mention one or two hobbies or achievements and demonstrate how these have helped you to develop useful skills than to attempt to list everything that interests you. Think carefully about which of your hobbies are relevant. The short, rushed sentence about being a football fan can be taken out completely as it is not relevant to the application.

Paragraph four: Refined

Here the applicant mentions only those hobbies that can be justified as relevant to their application. Remember that any hobbies involving attention to detail or hand-eye co-ordination are relevant to dentists, e.g. cooking, artwork, mechanics. Details are given as to how involvement in the Duke of Edinburgh award has helped them to develop and mature, showing the applicant to be a well-rounded person. This paragraph points to the contributions the student may make to the university community.

Concluding paragraph: Draft

No concluding paragraph has been given.

Concluding paragraph: Refined

'In conclusion, I consider myself a hardworking and well-rounded student and I look forward to making full use of the opportunities available to me at university.'

Concluding paragraph: Draft

A concluding paragraph is essential in order to leave the reader with a positive impression of your application and prevent the Personal Statement tailing off.

Concluding paragraph: Refined

The start of this sentence gives a hint that the Personal Statement is nearly finished, giving the reader time to reconsider the points the applicant has made. This is not the time to introduce new information so this section must be short, but it is important to summarise your key qualities and enthusiasm for future study.

Key points

The 'draft' and 'refined' versions of this fictitious example are presented in order to illustrate the principles underpinning the preparation of a compelling Personal Statement.

Your Personal Statement must describe **you**; **your** personal qualities, **your** enthusiasms, **your** strengths.

Make sure the material you present in your Personal Statement really does convince the reader that you have a very good idea of what you are getting into, that studying Dentistry is right for you, **and** that you are right for the dental profession.

Chapter 7

Personal Statement examples for applying to Dental School

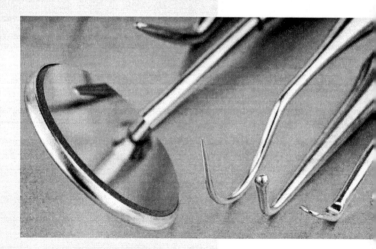

Personal Statement examples for applying to Dental School

Example 1

My motivation to study Dentistry came from frequent childhood visits to the dentist; an asymmetrical midline, caused by uneven numbers of teeth on my maxilla and mandible, led me to have braces fitted, and I will also need future bridgework to replace two missing adult teeth. This initial glimpse into the world of dentistry inspired me to undertake work placements with various dentists, where I discovered a genuine passion to pursue a dental career. Dentistry combines scientific application with manual dexterity and a level of patient contact unrivalled in many other professions. This amalgamation of skills interests me greatly and I feel that I could make a valuable contribution to the field.

I worked hard and studied independently to achieve excellent grades across my GCSE subjects, an achievement which expresses my love for learning, and which I have been able to carry over into my A levels. I am also aware that studying Dentistry requires independent study and the ability to face new challenges. At university I am particularly looking forward to learning about oral disease, having spent a week working in a microbiology lab, but am most looking forward to learning the clinical aspects of dentistry, including dealing with real patients and performing restorative surgeries such as fillings.

Through work experience placements, I have been able to gain an excellent insight into the challenges of a career in dentistry. Through shadowing an NHS dentist for four weeks, and spending a week of my summer holiday shadowing a dentist in Dubai, I learned about the various types of fillings, as well as the importance of good communication with patients. Watching the

---

nurse support the dentist by preparing impressions and fillings highlighted the necessity for teamwork, and by using suction during a scaling I was able to gain a true appreciation of the nurse's role in even a simple procedure. By talking to the dentists, I also had the opportunity to discuss issues ranging from cross-contamination to their views on Lord Darzi's reforms and their impact on the dental profession as a whole. During a week at the Microbiology Government Laboratory, I was responsible for preparing colonies of bacteria on agar plates and utilising quantitative polymerase chain reaction, developing my ability to keep a steady hand, whilst four days in Nottingham with Medlink gave me the opportunity to write a paper on nanotechnology; the issues I raised on tissue regeneration were published and can be viewed on the Medlink website. I volunteer weekly at Mencap, where I assist the elderly and people with various genetic disorders in participating in a range of activities.

At school, involvement in the Young Enterprise scheme as the Assistant Marketing Director helped me to develop my communication skills as part of a team and as a leader. Becoming a prefect has given me the responsibility of sharing advice with younger students, assisting in a year 8 class once a week and having a positive influence on their future. As an avid table tennis player I have been a sports leader at a local primary school, where I planned ideas and put them into motion with effective results. I have also coached both youngsters and people older than myself, requiring a balance of patience and the ability to handle people with different personalities. More recently I have started playing piano and I am also able to knit, pastimes which allow me to develop excellent manual dexterity and good concentration, both essential qualities in studying Dentistry.

Through my academic and work experiences, I feel that I have developed the necessary skills and knowledge to succeed in dentistry. I am passionate about pursuing such a rewarding and challenging career, and the Dentistry degree is my first step to achieving my ambitions.

Example 2

My passion for Biology and Chemistry has been fundamental to my choice of university courses, leading me naturally towards a career in dentistry and the sciences. Enthusiasm for discovery and understanding of biological processes influenced my selection of A level subjects, which I find challenging and rewarding. For my success at GCSE, I was awarded the St. Mary's Perpetual Shield and achieved first place in Biology and joint third in Additional Mathematics. I have completed the 'Application of Number' Key Skill to level three and competed in Mathematique Sans Frontieres in which my school won first place in the NEELB area.

My first true experience of dentistry was when I broke my front teeth and I am forever grateful for the patience and craftsmanship which restored the stumps to normality. Over the following months I was fascinated by the restoration process and this interest progressed, leading to a work placement in a dental surgery where I was able to regularly shadow a practising dentist. This provided opportunities to discuss many aspects of the profession including promotion of oral health, infection control and observation of a wide range of procedures, such as simple fillings, root canal fillings, restoration of acid damaged teeth and innovative techniques such as the use of a rubber dam to keep the teeth dry. It was evident that the dentist, hygienist and dental nurses communicated well and worked as a team. I witnessed the anxiety of patients and the need to develop a trusting relationship with them. Dentistry appeals to me because it demands a wide range of skills, from the interaction with patients to performing procedures which require attention to detail and accuracy. From my personal experience, the ability to restore patients' teeth to allow them to eat, look well and regain their confidence would be a very satisfying career.

For two summers, I volunteered to work in a hospital laboratory, where my main tasks were to assemble a blood culture collection kit and portering duties. From this I learnt to be precise, follow instructions, to be timely at completing the tasks and to communicate with the support services. Using my IT skills, I collated the data to assess the impact of introducing the kit. Working part-time in a local shop has taught me the importance of communication, punctuality, reliability and calmness under pressure. I have gained leadership experience as a school prefect, with the responsibility of helping at formal functions and acting as an ambassador for the school. Involvement in various charity fund raising events, such as completing the Concern 24-hour fast, enabled me to help those less fortunate than myself. Completion of a Deaf Awareness course has extended my communication skills. Computer games and model building have developed my innovativeness, hand-eye co-ordination, accuracy and manual dexterity. Being keen on strategy games, I coach younger club members, thereby improving my leadership and problem solving abilities, whilst membership of a tennis club has enhanced my teamwork skills. I enjoy piano playing and I am preparing for the Grade 3 Trinity College London examinations.

Dentistry attracts me because it is intellectually challenging and requires manual dexterity in a caring environment. Through my experiences, I have matured into a dedicated, diligent, self-motivated, caring person with good interpersonal skills. I am determined and committed to becoming a valued member of this profession, which plays a vital role in society.

Example 3

After completing my GCSE work experience at a dental practice, my childhood dream developed before my eyes into a real, tangible career choice that I would choose to pursue with enthusiasm and determination throughout my A level course. Whilst at the practice I observed how a single handed NHS surgery runs and experienced first-hand how the dentist interacts with the patients. Fuelled by the rewarding experiences at the practice, I spent the summer break after my AS level exams at a corporate practice while they were switching from NHS to private dental care. Whilst at the corporate clinic I was able to observe a wide range of dentists and realised how different dentists can be. During this time I also worked as a receptionist which enlightened me as to a very different perspective into the world of dentistry. Dealing with very different tasks such as appointments and administration enabled me to see the full extent of the work needed to run a dental practice whilst also enhancing my interpersonal skills. Also at this time, due to the switch from the NHS to a private 'Denplan' scheme, I was witness to the moral grounds for changing and how some patients benefited from the switch, whilst others did not.

I have always taken great pleasure in making a difference to other people's lives; I cared for an elderly man for seven years and was very sad when he died last year. I see being a dentist in much the same light; I have the chance to really better the health of another human being and this excites me in a way that no other potential profession ever has. Indeed, dentistry became particularly appealing to me when my sister's teeth were saved by a dental surgeon after a car crash last February; without the dentist, she would have had to deal with a disfigured jaw and false teeth. A dentist does, after all, deal with cosmetic issues as well as healthcare, and seeing my sister's face when she saw her teeth were not destroyed was one of the best moments of my life.

Dentistry involves dealing with people in a professional manner and keeping them calm when they are distressed. I feel I would be very good at this because of my ability to empathise with people. I developed this skill whilst on a three-day course in peer mentoring which involved dealing with distressed people by looking at and interpreting their body language, and changing our own accordingly. This is undoubtedly a skill that I will find very useful as a dentist. I have learnt how to prioritise and manage a larger workload throughout this year along with developing my self-discipline and organisational skills. My main interests are music and sport. I listen to music in order to relax, which allows me to get a sense of perspective on what events have occurred during the day. I play badminton, basketball, table tennis, football and have recently taken up tennis. Playing sport allows me to exercise my competitive edge in a healthy way and helps promote team play and the ability to handle pressure.

Looking to the future, I would love to own my own practice. The ability to help people in need is something that appeals so much to me, and becoming a dentist would provide me with tremendous job satisfaction.

Example 4

Over several years I have developed a keen curiosity about the medical environment, reading relevant articles and watching medical documentaries whenever possible. Since childhood I have also had a passion for making intricate models, and repairing things in my grandfather's workshop. After extensive work experience, I have concluded that a career in dentistry will allow me to combine my compassionate nature and aptitude for science with hands-on creative work.

Two months' work experience at my father's dental practice has allowed me to observe surgical and restorative dentistry, along with cosmetic and implant work. I was struck by the effect dental work can have on a person's well-being, by giving someone the confidence to smile again or using bridgework and implants to allow people to chew food. My father has patients who have been with him for decades, even coming from overseas for treatment, and I would love to be in a position to inspire such trust and respect. At his practice I also worked with the hygienist and receptionists, giving me a rounded view of the running of a practice. In addition, I have shadowed a local GP for three days, and spent a week with an Orthopaedic Consultant at a hospital. During this placement I spent time in consultations and surgery, and in A&E, which has given me a taste of the pressures of working in an emergency environment. Shadowing David Gault, a leading plastic surgeon in Europe, I had the privilege of observing him over a twelve-hour shift, during consultations, meetings and theatre, as well as learning from clinical videos of various operations which he kindly lent to me. My work experiences have filled me with enthusiasm for the field I am entering. At university I am looking forward to studying anatomy and physiology and also to learning how the latest technologies can be used to repair broken teeth. Having observed the impact technological advances have had in improving veneers, inlays, onlays and implants, I am very excited about the future of dentistry and my possible role within it.

Voluntary work at a nursing home has shown me a different side to healthcare and allowed me to develop my interpersonal skills dealing with residents. As a waiter and kitchen assistant in a restaurant, I worked within a busy team of people of all ages and backgrounds, serving demanding customers, and taking orders from chefs and managers. My position within the Combined Cadet Force, where I have risen to the rank of sergeant, has been a significant factor in my personal development. Discipline, leadership and team-building exercises are the focus of our training, and I have learnt many useful life skills. As a qualified marksman I enjoy clay pigeon and pheasant shooting, which requires a steady hand and an eye for accuracy. At school I have made an active contribution to the community, taking the lead role in several dramatic and musical productions and acting as producer and director of lower school plays. Visiting developing countries has widened my perspective of life, highlighting the worldwide need for qualified medical personnel. I have also toured South Africa with my rugby club, am a brown belt in judo, and enjoy swimming, fishing and diving.

My ambition is to specialise in dental cosmetics, smile makeovers and veneers, as I have seen the immediate impact cosmetic work can have on a person's self-esteem. As an active and sociable student I feel I can offer the appropriate balance between intellectand interpersonal skills which is required when intruding on someone's personal space through providing oral care. I am completely dedicated to practising as a dentist, and I feel I have the skills and motivation to achieve this goal.

Example 5

Dentistry appeals to me as my ideal area of study, being not only mentally stimulating, but practically challenging. As a dentist I will have the opportunity to make a positive contribution to my local community, and as a genuine and caring person with the determination to succeed in my studies, I am committed to studying Dentistry.

Currently studying a Medical Biology degree, I have developed a strong foundation in scientific knowledge which will prove essential in studying Dentistry; through perseverance and hard work I hope to achieve at least a 2.1 in my current studies. I am particularly looking forward to studying further into pharmacology, anatomy and physiology, subjects I enjoyed studying during my current degree, and I feel that my current academic experience means that I am already prepared for many of the pressures of studying Dentistry. I have also been able to practise good time management and learnt how to meet deadlines, alongside the necessity to balance my studies with outside activities.

In order to confirm my passion for dentistry, I have undertaken a range of placements including working at a doctors' surgery and with a consultant pharmacist, though it was my placement at the dentist which ultimately stood out as it was challenging on many fronts. The dentist has to be able to interact with patients and staff, as well as possessing a focused mind and good practical ability for performing demanding procedures. These are qualities that I possess, and I feel that dentistry will be a challenging and stimulating course which plays to my strengths. I observed many procedures being performed such as endodontic therapy, fillings and tooth removal, and am sure that the dental practice environment would give me the sense of belonging and identity I am looking for in my work environment.

Outside of work and study, my voluntary activities have helped me to develop a range of transferable skills, including leadership, communication and interpersonal skills. Volunteering for the Royal Society of Chemistry I was involved in the 'RSC: Next Generation project', a collaboration between Further Education institutes in Yorkshire and Humber and the RSC which aims to encourage higher students to take up more science-based subjects by emphasising the more enjoyable elements of Chemistry. Leading a team of two others, I was responsible for overseeing activities such as the 'the sweet DNA workshop', which I managed and ran. Through such activities I have had the opportunity to work with both academics and students, improving my ability to communicate with a range of people. Alongside this I was a member of the DNA model World Record Breaking Team within my undergraduate physiological society, and have also worked on the 'Marvellous Microbes' workshop in the school centre at the Thackray Museum, where I helped youngsters to understand the importance of manual hygiene.

I appreciate the need to balance my work and study with leisure activities, and enjoy running, having held the cross-country record for my school. Playing football, badminton and cricket, alongside crocheting, has enabled me to improve my focus and co-ordination. I am also a student of Islam, and through dedicating time to studying the Qur'an and fasting during Ramadan, I have learnt discipline of both the mind and body.

Ultimately, my aim is to open my own NHS practice in the community in which I grew up, and the opportunity to study Dentistry at university is not one I take lightly. I am committed to succeeding in whatever I do and enjoy challenges; as such, I feel that I am prepared for this degree and will dedicate myself completely to excelling as a Dentistry student.

Example 6

I consider dentistry to be a form of art; where manual dexterity enables you to make a difference to people's lives. Since spending two weeks in a general NHS dental practice as part of my lower-school work experience, it has been my ambition in life to become a dentist. I feel that dentistry offers many challenges both 'hands-on' and intellectually.

To explore the opportunities a career in dentistry offers, I have spent the last two years working as a voluntary dental assistant in a local NHS practice. This experience has provided me with an invaluable insight into what is expected of a dentist. I was able to observe many dental procedures and the need for good interpersonal skills to relax the patient and ensure that they are aware of the procedure being performed. I was responsible for assisting the dentist in ensuring that everything was prepared correctly for each consultation whilst ensuring the needs of the patient were met.

As my A level studies have progressed I have particularly enjoyed learning about the human body, especially in relation to care and treatment. I look forward to furthering my knowledge of physiology and the complex nature of oral care and treatment. It is my intention, as part of my career as a dentist, to contribute to the intellectual understanding of dentistry by undertaking research in an appropriate area. This will enable me to embrace my keen interest in furthering my understanding in physiological processes. Having also spent the last year working in a local nursing home as a care assistant, I have found this experience highly rewarding and it has greatly improved my ability to interact with people. My responsibilities have included preparing meals, maintaining the hygiene and well-being of the elderly residents and interacting with them to keep them mentally stimulated. Caring for the elderly has cemented my intention to follow a career where I can interact with people, make a difference to their lives and alleviate any suffering.

I consider myself to be a motivated and outgoing individual both within and outside of school. One of my greatest achievements at school was being awarded the 'Most Improved Pupil' award in Year 11 in recognition of the vast improvement in my progress. I enjoy playing the flute in the school orchestra and have achieved my Grade 6. Participating in team sports is very enjoyable and I have represented my Sixth Form in both hockey and netball. The responsibility of being a school prefect has developed my interpersonal skills through interacting with a variety of people.

It is my intention to embrace everything that studying Dentistry at university has to offer. As a committed, motivated and enthusiastic dental student I will be able to contribute to university life in a variety of ways, both academically and in the extra-curricular sense. Through successfully completing my degree in Dentistry I will be able to realise my dream of following my chosen career path and contributing to the dental profession as a whole.

Example 7

Some people say 'people only become a dentist if they cannot become a doctor!' However, I disagree with this statement profusely. Working as a dentist encompasses a wide range of skills and notions that you do not find in any other field of treatment provision. Where else are you faced with such varied tasks ranging from interacting with patients to performing procedures which require exquisite attention to detail and accuracy? In my opinion, a career in dentistry offers an individual both intellectual and manual challenges which I would relish immensely.

My ambition to become a dentist stems from my experiences gained whilst working in an NHS dental practice as an assistant. I have spent the last 18 months gaining an invaluable insight into what is expected from a dentist in the day-to-day running of a busy practice. Through talking to patients, I have learnt what is required in terms of interpersonal contact and have enjoyed interacting with a range of people. I am particularly attracted to this field due to the diverse nature of dentistry and the opportunity to specialise in fields ranging from orthodontics to cosmetic dentistry. Other work experience I have carried out has included working as a volunteer in my local shelter for the homeless. My responsibilities have included interacting with the public and providing food and blankets to the people staying at the shelter. This experience has been very rewarding and has reinforced my desire to work in an environment where I can interact with people and make a difference to their lives.

At school I have enjoyed success in both my academic and extra-curricular activities. Through studying Human Biology I have come to understand the complex nature of the human body and would like to further my understanding and knowledge of this at university level. I am an active member of the school debating team which has improved my confidence by speaking to large numbers of people. I am part of the school football and rugby teams where

I have experienced success in reaching the last round of the regional finals for both sports. I am also a keen musician and enjoy playing the piano and guitar in a local rock band, successfully playing at a number of local venues. My hobby of painting models, ranging from cars to aeroplanes, has enhanced my manual dexterity which is an essential requirement in dentistry.

I would describe myself as a motivated and committed individual who intends to take advantage of the wide range of opportunities that studying at university has to offer. Through studying Dentistry I will be able to fulfil my lifetime ambition of becoming a dentist and successfully managing my own practice. A career in dentistry will provide me with the ongoing challenges of personal development which I desire, enable me to have regular daily contact with patients, and provide me with the opportunity to make a difference to people's lives.

Example 8

Dentistry appeals to me as it combines a high level of patient interaction with the opportunity to use practical skills and scientific knowledge in order to improve people's oral health. During my A level studies I have enjoyed working with a variety of materials and using logical analysis to make scientific evaluations and I now wish to make use of these skills to make a positive contribution to people's wellbeing.

Whilst studying Chemistry and Biology at A level, I have particularly enjoyed learning about human physiology and cell structure and I am keen to develop this with the study of all aspects of prevention, alleviation and treatment of oral health problems and injuries at university. I am also particularly looking forward to spending clinical placements involved in patient treatment as I feel this will be the best way to understand the skills needed for effective clinical practice and to put the theory into context. Having attended several pre-med courses I have gained an insight into the content and structure of the initial dentistry training. These courses have confirmed that it is the medical science and procedures relating to oral health and the positive impact good oral health can have on an individual's life which particularly interests me.

Work experience shadowing a dentist for three weeks at an NHS dental surgery has given me an insight into the day-to-day running of a practice and the qualities required of a successful dentist. My observations included a wide range of treatments from a simple filling to more complex surgical procedures. I found that one of the most important qualities required is to have good communication skills. This is utilised in helping to put patients at ease, discussing treatment plans and thereby ensuring informed consent, and in working as an integral part of a dynamic team. I also made the most of the opportunity to discuss my career and training options with practising dentists. The almost limitless scope for further enhancement of my career and professional expertise offered by dentistry particularly appeals to me. Through two one-week work experience placements in a hospital, and an ongoing position as a volunteer ward assistant, I have widened my understanding of the healthcare system and developed my interpersonal skills with staff, patients and families. Through my ongoing volunteering at a residential home and previous community service at a primary school, a nursery and a play scheme, I have gained valuable experience of communicating with both children and older people, developing my confidence and maturity at the same time.

At school I have developed my leadership skills through heading the Muslim assembly and taking part in the charity committee and I look forward to contributing similarly to the university community. I also work voluntarily at an Oxfam shop once a week, and have completed 200 hours of service as a Millennium Volunteer. In my leisure time I enjoy playing on the school rounders team, as well as playing tennis and boxing. For the past two years I have been competing in cross country running, for which I achieved a gold award, and taking lessons in karate, in which I have now reached red belt. I also attend classes in embroidery and sewing, which have utilised both my creativity and my dexterity.

In conclusion, I have taken care to thoroughly research dentistry as a career in order to make a well-informed choice about my future. My dental work experience has confirmed my enthusiasm and suitability for this career. I am fully committed to my ambition of running my own dental practice, and I feel I have the skills and motivation to achieve this goal.

Example 9

My ideal career is one that would include science, public healthcare, my own creative flair and hands-on challenges that involve a continually evolving subject. I know that there is no better career for me that would incorporate these more than dentistry. I have a firm belief that everyone deserves the right to a smile that they can be proud of and a dentist they can trust. My gifts in manual dexterity, spatial awareness and attention to detail are well-honed, and I look forward to building on these skills through studying Dentistry.

I am a recent graduate from the University of Liverpool; I achieved a BSc degree in Microbiology and was awarded the Honours Prize in the Microbiology/Biotechnology Department. During my degree I found myself drawn towards medical microbiology and found oral health modules and journals especially fascinating. My degree will benefit my career in dentistry via my understanding of communicable infectious diseases. I have now developed my study skills beyond their earlier levels and can approach dentistry with a maturity I could not have reached immediately following A level. The clinical content of the Dentistry course excites me the most, especially detection and treatment of diseases, and practising new techniques.

My aim in the future is to become a general Dental Practitioner and eventually own a practice. I would like to further my studies to eventually include cosmetic dental procedures in my range of treatments, which would provide more treatment options to my patients. I am aware that dental practice is also a business which requires strong leadership and financial management skills to make it a successful one. I believe my previous part-time work as a team leader has helped me to improve these skills. This role involved delegating tasks, motivating individuals, and being an approachable person. I have also spent long hours in microbiology labs working on delicate procedures and moulding tiny intricate models from many materials, thus improving my manual dexterity. This skill has been enhanced further by regularly playing the clarinet from the age of nine.

I have had the opportunity to shadow a wide range of professionals within dentistry, including a private dental surgeon, NHS dentist, Endodontist, Orthodontist, dental hygienist and dental nurse. I was able to practise everyday jobs and I also scrubbed in to observe an implant surgery, which included me holding a camera in a patient's mouth and handling sterile equipment. I have also had lengthy discussions with undergraduate dental students to gain an idea about their experiences and the pressures they face. I also spent a year in the A&E department of Aintree Hospital where I learnt how to become more empathetic and reassuring towards patients. Moreover, at school, I mentored pupils with learning disabilities which helped me to explain complicated facts in a way that is easier for others to understand.

I have achieved my Bronze and Silver Duke of Edinburgh awards and have almost completed the Gold award. In 2003 I also completed a month long expedition to Costa Rica, with 'Team Challenge'. These experiences have helped me develop my interpersonal skills and understand that both leadership and teamwork are needed for success in challenging situations. I was a committee member of the university skiing club, which included managing expenditures of the club and organising trips and socials. I also rowed for the university team, including at Women's Henley 2008; I would like to continue with these commitments at university. My activities show that I am able to keep my life in a good balance, whilst learning to prioritise my academics.

In summation, I am a well balanced, enthusiastic individual who is an ideal candidate for studying Dentistry and I am eager to commit myself to this highly respected field.

Example 10

My interest in dentistry began from my childhood experience of wearing a retainer. The effect that this had on the formation and presentation of my teeth made me aware that dentistry is not merely a medical science but is a fulfilling profession that incorporates a myriad of skills ranging from creating and ensuring a patients' self confidence to the delivery of oral education to all types of people. My own family dentist had always impressed on me the importance of oral hygiene, so I have developed meticulous techniques. It is my ambition to train to become a dentist and have a positive effect on people's lives.

My commitment and enthusiasm for studying Dentistry is evident in the work experience I have been undertaking. I currently work shadow at a general dental practice every Thursday for three hours. This has given me a valuable insight to the holistic nature of dentistry. I have gained experience of the work of dentists, dental nurses, dental hygienists and therapists. Working within this environment has consolidated my desire to study Dentistry whilst developing many work related skills. I understand the importance of working in a team as well as the need to demonstrate leadership and vision. I also believe that it is imperative to be able to communicate effectively with colleagues and patients.

I have not only gained work-related skills through my work experience at a dental practice. I have also developed excellent customer service experience through my part-time job at Sainsbury's. I am used to liaising effectively with others as part of a multidisciplinary team, and working in a wide range of environments. I have to demonstrate the professionalism and commitment required to deliver the highest standards of service. I also work independently, strictly following departmental guidelines and other relevant procedures and am partly responsible for ensuring the availability and safe storage of stock, including reordering as necessary. It has also provided me with some financial independence. This, I feel, is an important aspect to university life.

Within my academic environment, I am a self-motivated and mature pupil active in many aspects of school life. As a prefect, I have enjoyed showing prospective parents and pupils around the school. This created an opportunity for me to work with primary school children. Becoming a mentor to primary school pupils enabled me to ensure their smooth transition to high school. I have also become involved in the school theatrical productions, designing and making the background sets and props. This has been excellent for my creative and artistic skills. As a member of the school football and rugby team, I believe in team work and the desire to achieve. Lastly, I am furthering my creativity by learning to play the guitar.

As a determined and driven individual I feel I have a good understanding of the complexities and challenges that lie ahead as student of Dentistry. I would relish the varying teaching and learning techniques employed in Dentistry courses from simulated patient models to more traditional lectures. As a well organised and prepared person during my current studies, part-time job and work shadowing, I have been able to prioritise my tasks. This can easily be transferred to a university environment. My principles as a person are commitment, dedication, enthusiasm and communication.

Lastly, I view dentistry as a vocation. I envisage myself concentrating in Orthodontistry as a career path and I believe in a holistic approach. I would relish the opportunity to study the subject at your institution.

Example 11

The biggest challenge I have had to face is writing this statement in a way that fully encapsulates how much the study of Dentistry means to me. Being a naturally hard working, friendly and committed person, with a great drive and enthusiasm to reach my goals, I believe that I have much to offer as a future dentist.

Currently in my final year of my BEng Dental Materials course, I have learnt a lot about the career and clinical applications of treatment materials. I carried out some lab work with a PhD student who was testing a new material for the adhesion of tooth filling. I found it very interesting, managing to get some lab experience and to also see some clinical application. My degree offered me the chance to study a module in Maxillofacial Anatomy. I thoroughly enjoyed it and wanted to learn more so I decided to carry out some work experience to show me what medical applications occur within Maxillofacial Surgery. I now work for a charity called Saving Faces. I assisted in carrying out a national survey for facial injury cases dealt with by Oral and Maxillofacial Surgery Departments and A&E. I was taught a lot about how the charity benefits people with facial injuries and mouth/throat cancer. I learnt that reconstructive surgery can make many patients happy as a facial disfigurement is something they are reminded of every day. Also, having undertaken a wide variety of work experience in the field I have a very open view to the world of dentistry.

I like that every day is a new day. Being a sociable person I enjoy the idea of meeting new people and having new cases to deal with. I understand that it is a branch of medicine and that health and appearance of teeth can influence someone's life. My first work experience in the field was at a community dental surgery where I saw a lot of patients who were mentally handicapped or had an extreme fear of visiting the dentist. It was good to see how the dentist dealt with stressful situations. This made me realise the important of patience and keeping calm. During my time at private dental surgeries I saw a lot of different types of dental materials being used and it was exciting to see the restorative materials being clinically applied. They carried out various types of treatments including Orthodontics, Endodontology, restorative treatments and preventative treatment. The most interesting treatment I saw take place was aesthetic gum treatment. I also found the implantology fascinating. The second clinic was based on aesthetic treatments; mostly whitening of the teeth. During my time in Africa I worked on two projects: a government funded surgery and at an outreach project in local villages and orphanages. During the outreach programme, which was a great team working experience, I helped educate and treat those with poor finance and poor oral education. I also climbed Mt Kilimanjaro to raise money for Saving Faces and the British Dental Health Foundation.

At university I am excited about studying oral diseases and in greater depth about maxillofacial anatomy. I realise that there will be added pressures but they can be overcome by using the skills I have gained by studying my current degree. Skills such as organisation, time management and planning can all help reduce pressure. My degree has taught me to keep calm under pressure and when I do think it is getting too much I go to the gym to unwind. I will also make an effort to keep my life balanced so I can still enjoy my hobbies and social life. Long term, I would like to practise as a dentist and specialise in Oral Surgery.

Example 12

For a long time, I was torn between the study of Medicine and the study of Dentistry, as both of these disciplines have always been at the forefront of my career aspirations. They are both professions centred around making a real difference to the health of another individual, and what could be more important and worthwhile than that? It was after much research into the different areas of medicine that I found myself leaning towards dentistry. I was presented with many questions about the history of dentistry and dental care, and ultimately oral health as a whole; how were oral operations carried out and how has oral care developed over the years?

At the start of my lower Sixth Form, I felt that work experience in a health clinic would help me in deciding my future career. Here I had the opportunity to discuss all aspects of the medical profession with the GP. After this, I was fortunate enough to attend the local dental practice for further work experience. Whilst there, I discovered a great deal about the demands of the job, forming a realistic opinion about what a career in dentistry is all about. I also discovered many aspects of the career that I had previously not known about. These aspects excited and interested me, and from then on I decided to focus my academic studies on Dentistry.

Towards the end of my lower Sixth Form, I started a 12-month placement doing voluntary work at the local Dental Surgeon's office on a weekly basis. My duties include assisting the nurses in their work, where I get to do a lot of hands-on tasks. A vital part of this voluntary scheme is interacting with the patients, which has improved my interpersonal skills and I have learnt to communicate effectively with a diverse group of people and deal with difficult and sometimes emotional situations.

This July, I was a successful applicant for a community project at school and selected to work with a group of other students to form a peer listening service for younger pupils. Formal training was given by educational psychologists and during this time I acquired many skills such as listening and problem solving. With these skills I can help others in need and also apply them to life in general, particularly the dental profession; it can often be terribly frightening to attend the dentist, and I'd like to think that I am capable of reassuring and comforting patients.

In my spare time I like to play badminton for my own relaxation and attend the local gym to keep fit. Reading is one of my hobbies and I have read many works of classic literature by authors such as Austen, Hardy, Shakespeare and Dickens. Outside of school, I am continuing to learn French as I have always had an intense interest in this language. To keep updated with the latest advances in science, I read New Scientist regularly.

I enjoy working under my own steam but I believe I can also work as part of an effective team. I hope one day to work in a practice where I can use some of my personal qualities to serve the needs of a local community. I am methodical, able to undertake precise tasks and assimilate detailed information quickly. I am also diligent, hard-working and determined to succeed. I am therefore very well suited to a career in dentistry and look forward to being an active member of your institution.

Example 13

I started to consider a career in dentistry before my first degree; however, I felt that I would do more justice to the course, and to the career, if I had the benefit of maturity and highly developed study skills. Though Engineering often helps people indirectly, I want to enter into a career where I can help people directly, and through interacting with patients during my work experience and seeing the benefits first-hand, I am now keen to study Dentistry in order to progress onto a career as a skilled dentist.

The achievement of my first degree in Engineering was a very proud moment for me and I feel that my academic ability has seen a drastic improvement throughout my studies. Studying for four years has given me an appreciation of the rigours of a long university course, and I have a good idea of what it's like to train towards acquiring skills in a specific vocation. One of the areas that I enjoyed at college concerned materials and how they react when forces are applied to them, and I am keen to study the most recent trends in biomaterials, biomimetics and biophotonics. During my degree I was able to develop good planning, a disciplined approach and the ability to meet deadlines and adapt quickly. I also enjoy tasks involving a high degree of manual dexterity, and am excited about the lifelong learning involved in dentistry.

Observing in two different dental practices has enabled me to gain an insight into the treatment of NHS and private patients during a wide range of procedures, including root canals, crowns, and an extraction which involved sectioning. One of the surgeries used cutting-edge technology, including animations to show procedures to patients, whilst the other surgery was very old-fashioned; however, the skill of the dentists and manner towards their patients was equally impressive in both practices, and I learned the importance of discussing procedures clearly with every patient. I also spent a day with a restorative dentist and Maxillofacial Surgeons at St Richard's Hospital in Chichester, where I learnt that the emphasis was on achieving the best possible compromise for the patient and decisions were made on the balance between risk and benefit for each procedure. In one particular case, a patient who had undergone extensive reconstructive surgery after a car accident was not completely happy with his bite; the potential dangers of further surgery led the surgeon to discourage the patient from going ahead, highlighting the kinds of decisions dentists have to make, often under a great deal of pressure.

Working for Devon County Council requires that I attend meetings and give presentations. I am expected to deputise for my line manager in his absence and deal with software problems as they occur, developing my ability to work accurately under pressure. I possess highly developed IT skills, with a working knowledge of word-processing, spreadsheets and presentation software as well as software packages for 2D and 3D modelling animation, finite element analysis (FEA) and other computer programs. Outside of work, I took responsibility for 15 boys aged 14–15 at Camp America, alongside three other counsellors; I had to balance being approachable with exercising my authority when necessary and this, combined with volunteering in a care home for the elderly, means that I am comfortable communicating with people of all ages and temperaments.

I am committed to personal development and would love to keep training and absorbing new techniques throughout my working life. I believe that my drive and desire to succeed in the field of dentistry, as well as my years of prior experience studying in an establishment of higher learning, makes me an ideal candidate to study Dentistry.

Example 14

While I knew that my future career would involve the sciences, it was during a work placement at my village practice that I was introduced to the broad range of abilities, knowledge and responsibilities a dentist has. An implant operation was of special interest to me as it helped me realise how much dentistry is involved with the patient's general well-being and quality of life. I enjoyed my two weeks helping in the surgery and this sparked my interest in dentistry as a career.

With a view to studying Dentistry at university, I arranged to shadow a Senior Oral Surgeon at Nobles Hospital, after which there was no doubt in my mind that I had chosen the right career. My time there has provided me with an invaluable insight through the observation of surgical procedures such as an apicectomy and a biopsy. This experience has helped me understand the need for calm and reassuring communication skills when dealing with anxious patients. I spent a further week at my village practice during which I was able to discuss with the qualified dentists the commitment needed for a career in dentistry. Additional work placements have been organised with the hospital to extend my knowledge and experience.

At Sixth Form College, I have found the practical elements of my science subjects of particular interest and enjoy using new equipment and materials as the course work progresses. At Dental School, I am looking forward to understanding the techniques and mechanics behind implants and more complex surgical procedures. While considering my university options, I attended an Army 'Look at Life Course' with the Lancaster Regiment which focused on leadership and teamwork. I was able to use this experience in my role as Managing Director with Young Enterprise. Working at the bank has developed my financial awareness as well as giving me the necessary skills and confidence to deal with a wide range of customers.

I also manage my own rock band and run a weekend gardening business. Balancing these activities with my A level study has required a responsible nature and good organisational skills. This experience will help support me through university life and studies.

Competing in rifle shooting competitions has needed both determination and a disciplined practice regime as I have progressed to a high standard, hoping one day to represent the Isle of Man in the Commonwealth Games. To keep fit I swim once a week with the local club. Rugby is also a favourite sport and I play for both the school team and a local club, travelling to England to compete in matches.

I enjoy reading and spending time with my friends. Music is important to me socially and for relaxation. This includes playing the piano up to Grade 3 and the electric guitar as well singing and playing with the band for the school and at social events. I also enjoy taking part in musicals, school plays and local pantomimes. International travel with my family and meeting people from all walks of life has broadened my outlook. I give time to the community through helping the Red Cross and fundraising for Samaritans.

I have confidence in my decision to become a dentist. Having thoroughly researched my options and undertaken related work experience, I am fully committed to a career in dentistry. My ultimate goal is to become an Oral Surgeon and I am looking forward to the challenges and opportunities of university life.

Example 15

Following directly in the footsteps of many family members, I am experienced in the nature of dentistry and the responsibilities, tasks and skills involved in becoming a dentist.

I am currently studying Biology, Chemistry and Mathematics. I feel that this specialised subject combination would be very useful for dentistry, as it would provide a good command of the dental discipline and also good communication skills for understanding and dealing with patients. I particularly enjoy the practical side to my Chemistry lessons, and such a good grounding in science will prepare me especially well for the strong science aspect of the Dentistry course. I am particularly good with my hands, having built model aeroplanes for seven years. This will undoubtedly help with the difficulties of working with teeth in such a small space as the human mouth.

I have worked at three different dental practices. These experiences have proven to be very informative and have reinforced that dentistry is definitely the profession for me, heightening my enthusiasm. The work is dynamic and challenging and involves interacting with many different types of people. At one of the practices I was given the opportunity to shadow an Orthodontist. This has made me very keen to learn more about the various specialist fields available in dentistry. I have worked as a classroom assistant in a primary school, so I can appreciate the difficulties of calming children enough to have dental procedures carried out on them. I feel that my experience with the Orthodontist, combined with my experiences with children, furnished me well in terms of my ability to empathise with and calm patients with anxiety.

I participate in various extra-curricular activities. I have gained the Junior Sports Leader Award in recognition of my work as a sportswoman. I play netball, basketball, badminton and tennis. I also enjoy singing and writing song lyrics. I have participated in many performance art events. Last year I sang on stage to a crowd of over 3,000 people, which I found challenging but very rewarding. At university I hope to continue to add to my extra curricular achievements.

Over the years my range of skills have increased through my work experience, leisure activities and studying. I am, for example, an excellent communicator who works well individually and in a team. I am also quite creative as I love putting new ideas into practice. I am confident in always trying to achieve my best possible result and have a bright, extrovert, personality; I am friendly, I always approach everything with enthusiasm, and I am always ready to contribute.

I would be extremely grateful to be given the opportunity to become a dentist. I feel this profession holds such an essential and vital role in society and I believe my dedication to this career, and passion for helping others, will allow me to one day become a valued member of this competitive and demanding profession.

Example 16

Throughout my school years I have sought a challenging and rewarding profession that would satisfy my passion for science and the need to express my artistic and dextrous abilities, whilst allowing me to work closely with people to make a positive impact in their lives. Frequent visits to the dentist for orthodontic treatment triggered my fascination for dentistry and fuelled my aspirations to pursue a career in this demanding yet satisfying profession. I have a strong desire to not only improve the health and wellbeing of people, but to embark on a life-long experience of learning and development in which I can constantly improve my knowledge and practical skills and embrace technological advancements in clinical dentistry.

My work experience at four dental practices has further reinforced my determination to study Dentistry. I was privileged to be able to shadow and assist dental practitioners; carrying out suction on patients undergoing procedures, sterilising instruments and developing x-rays. While I observed an Orthodontist, a Periodontist and an Oral Surgeon as they performed procedures such as fillings, root canal treatments, extractions, implants, flap surgery and fitting of braces, I was struck by the immense patience, attention to detail and precision with which this intricate work was carried out. I learned, too, the importance of responsive communication with the patients and derived great satisfaction from being able to reassure and calm nervous patients before and during their treatment. My work as a dental receptionist during the summer months expanded my interpersonal, management and teamwork skills and gave me a valuable insight into the effective functioning of a busy dental practice. Teamwork is an important part of my voluntary and charity activities as well, particularly my involvement with Saint Francis Hospice where staff, volunteers and families work together to ensure the best quality of life for terminally ill patients. Having travelled to India and witnessed poverty and hardship, I feel strongly that I want to continue to help others wherever possible. I am a member of the volunteer team at a school for children with special needs, where I enjoy taking responsibility for mentoring children, helping them to achieve their goals, providing support and responding to their individual needs. I plan to expand my volunteer work in my gap year by taking part in teaching projects in India and Nepal.

As a sociable and practical person I found the responsibility of running clubs and activities at school immensely rewarding. Sewing and embroidery is a long standing hobby so I organised a school textiles club in which I could develop my manual dexterity and teach other members to create intricate patchwork and embroidered pieces. My passion for science and maths inspired me to run a science club and an economics club in which I could mentor younger students in areas in which they were struggling, and get involved in lively debates concerning current controversial issues. Being a member of the school magazine was a great opportunity to expand my organisational and teamwork skills to regularly produce interesting and informative articles against a strict deadline.

I am a committed, determined and hardworking person looking forward to the responsibility and challenges of studying at university. I am confident I will be able to balance the academic demands of the course with social and relaxing activities such as badminton and yoga, and will be organised and enthusiastic in my approach to my studies. I am fully aware of the lengthy and demanding nature of the course but my commitment and motivation convinces me I will achieve my ambition and make a positive contribution to the field of dentistry.

Example 17

Dentistry appeals to me as it combines a high level of patient interaction with the opportunity to use practical skills and scientific knowledge to solve real life problems. In my first degree I have enjoyed working with a variety of materials and using logical analysis to make scientific evaluations and I now wish to make use of these skills to make a positive contribution to people's health.

My degree has given me a useful background to the modules on pharmacology and biochemistry. As I enjoy practical work, I am particularly interested in the hands on study of dental biomaterial. Completing a demanding degree involved managing large volumes of information and prioritising high workloads with strict deadlines. During my individual and group research, for example, my final year project on cytotoxic drugs in cancer chemotherapy, I have presented my conclusions via a range of media. I am also confident using IT software such as model building programmes and advanced data banks.

During work experience in an Orthodontist's practice, I was able to observe a range of procedures and consultations. I enjoyed the opportunity to interact with a diverse range of patients and to learn from the healthcare team. I have also arranged a shadowing placement at a Dental GP's surgery which will widen my experience and allow me to learn more about the breadth of a dentist's work. I am particularly excited by the prospect of spending three years involved in patient treatment as I feel this will be the best way to understand clinical practices and to put theory into context.

As a Play Leader I have experience of communicating with people of all ages, as well as supervising primary age children and organising activities such as coach trips, and plays to which parents were invited. My customer service jobs, including silver service waiting, and barman at two Lanzarote night clubs, have given me confident interpersonal skills. Currently I work within a team of night assistants at an Asda store. This is a pressurised job as our role is to maintain stock levels throughout the Christmas rush and January sales. For several months I have been an adult volunteer with the Air Cadets and this has supplemented the skills I developed during a recent Royal Navy potential officer course focusing on leadership and management.

Membership of the Rowing Club, a university seven-a-side football team, and a local football team has allowed me to build on my teamwork skills and provided a balance to my academic studies. Participating in the Welsh Society allowed me to learn more about my cultural heritage and meet many new people. As a mature student I envisage myself making a positive contribution to the student community, supporting younger students with Chemistry, IT or problems adjusting to university life. Since graduating, I have been teaching myself the guitar, and I continue to keep up to date with scientific developments through journals. I intend to gain useful experience during my gap year and am currently preparing for an interview in November for a position in a hospital cytology lab.

In conclusion, my maturity and experience has allowed me to make a well-informed choice about my future and will be of great assistance in allowing me to work to my full potential during my degree. My dental work experience has confirmed my enthusiasm and suitability for this career and I am fully committed to my ambition of running my own dental practice, as I feel I have the skills and motivation to achieve this goal.

Example 18

My interest in dentistry stems from a desire to follow a mentally challenging but creative and practical profession. Extensive work experience has confirmed my choice, particularly as it involves a high degree of patient interaction. In my opinion, a career in dentistry offers many challenges, both 'hands-on' and intellectually, which I would relish immensely. I feel I am able to undertake precise tasks methodically and assimilate detailed information quickly. I am also diligent, hard-working and determined to succeed.

Biology A level has been useful in providing me with a good understanding of the human anatomy and physiological processes. Chemistry involves a high degree of practical group research giving the challenge of incorporating the whole group's ideas into a final plan. I find the need for independent learning and problem solving in Mathematics invigorating, especially when several different approaches are needed before finding the answer. I look forward to studying a degree which will utilise my skills to implement practical techniques.

I attended several highly informative dentistry and health-related summer schools, which allowed me to try out practical tasks such as fitting braces onto a model as well as allowing me to gain insight into what a Dentistry degree entails. I organised work experience at a dental practice in Slough where I observed root canal treatment and extractions, and learnt about the differences between private and NHS work. Through discussions with the dentist, I realised the impact such a career can have on your personal life and was given advice about running my own practice. On a placement at a Referral Centre, I shadowed dentists performing oral surgery. I particularly noticed the need for a reassuring manner with patients, especially children, and the importance of effective communication and trust between the dental team and patients. Through performing tasks such as preparing beds, filing and making appointments, I had the opportunity to work with people from different cultural backgrounds and observe many different procedures.

Working in the Pathology & Haematology department of a hospital, I enjoyed practising testing procedures and techniques; however, I realised that I would prefer dealing with a patient all the way from consultation to the final evaluation, as in dentistry. I have also worked part-time in a busy restaurant on the till, serving customers, and in the pressurised environment of the kitchen, where I enjoyed being part of a team pulling together to achieve high results. Dealing with agitated customers and working to deadlines required the ability to cope under pressure. On joining a new Sixth Form, I enjoyed the opportunity to meet new friends and get involved in school life by assisting at Open Days and organising tours for parents. Attending Amnesty International each week has developed my confidence in sharing my ideas, organising new tasks, and obtaining our yearly objectives. Mentoring a year 11 pupil was a rewarding task, particularly when he achieved higher than expected GCSEs. The main outcome of these experiences was the dramatic improvement in my communicational skills. Outside school I play the dhol, with others, at cultural events which has given me self assurance when performing in front of large groups. I go jogging each morning and play in cricket and football teams during weekends, as well as organising tournaments. Attending religious festivals is a big part of my life and I help organise pool competitions and run the gym at my local gurdwara.

Having thoroughly researched my options I am fully committed to a career in dentistry. My ambition is to run my own practice and I feel I have the skills and motivation to succeed both at university and in my future career.

Chapter 3

Example 19

My determination to follow a career in healthcare was sparked when my grandfather developed a cancer that spread to the maxillary bone, presenting with a gum swelling that was spotted by a dentist. This experience highlighted the importance of the wider role of the dentist in providing important health screening for their patients, and studying Dentistry will develop both my understanding of, and suitability for, this role in the future.

My love of science stems from my naturally inquisitive character. My fascination for learning more about the body and how it works, and the impact of disease and illness, means that I am excited at the prospect of studying human anatomy and physiology. I am particularly looking forward to the 'hands on' aspects of the course as it really appeals to my practical nature and my love of manually fixing and assembling items. I feel that studying Economics at AS level and Business Studies at GCSE level has given me an insight into the economic and business aspects of running a dental practice. Meanwhile, I feel that being an avid reader with a passion to keep up-to-date with modern developments, and being fully conversant with a range of computer programs, has been vital in supporting me in my academic work.

My decision to apply to study Dentistry was reinforced by my work experience at a local dental surgery, where I was impressed by the manual dexterity and precision demonstrated by the dentists while constructing bridges, crowns and moulded dentures. I also have a keen interest in Maxillofacial Surgery and was given the opportunity to watch as the dentist glued moulded dentures onto implants inserted by the Maxillofacial Surgeon. Observing a dentist at work and discussing dentistry with him was a revealing and rewarding experience. Furthermore, I spent a few days at a local hospice which was another challenging and worthwhile experience, as speaking to patients with life limiting illness made me consider very carefully the way I interacted with people. It also offered me the chance to practise appropriate communication skills in an emotionally demanding environment.

Fulfilling roles that require me to take responsibility demonstrates my ability to rise to challenges and see tasks through to the end. At school I am currently the Senior Prefect for Charities, the treasurer of the common room committee and also hold the position of Head of House, where my naturally gregarious and sociable nature makes the job of organising and supporting charity events a rewarding pleasure. Running the school's Medical Society, and expanding the focus to dentistry also, is an achievement that I am proud of and has proved a success in giving it broader appeal, and pupils the opportunity to learn about both careers.

Involvement in sports has been an enduring passion; playing rugby for the school and football for a local club has improved my health and stamina, and importantly my teamwork skills. The process of training for the teams has required self-discipline and commitment, which I have demonstrated by consistent attendance and application within the sessions. I have used my sports experience to good effect by volunteering at sports events helping young children in various activities. This helped enhance my communication skills with a younger age group.

I will ensure that I make the most of the opportunities presented to me at university. Dentistry is a career in which I can combine my personal qualities of compassion and kindness with my love for applied Biomedical Sciences, enjoying practical work and interacting with people. Completing this degree is a goal that I am committed to achieving.

Example 20

As a qualified Paediatrician I wish to study Dentistry in order to work in the field of Oral Medicine. Maxillofacial Prosthetics is the area I particularly wish to work in and I feel the combination of medical and dental knowledge will give me the best possible preparation for this field.

My Medicine degree has given me a good understanding of most of the medical areas which feature in the Dentistry course. As I achieved the highest grade for almost every component of my course, and I have experience of degree level group research, presentations, and self-directed learning, I feel I am fully prepared for entering tertiary level study in this country. Once qualified, I am interested in researching the restoration of maxillofacial function and aesthetics in post-surgical and trauma patients, particularly that of intraoral acquired defects.

Whilst at university I was involved in the Student Union, helping and motivating young people in local colleges and other community settings and welcoming them to events at our university. Running campus tours and working with subject related groups, I enjoyed mixing with a wide range of people and developing my organisation and communication skills. At my future university I intend to be involved in the Students' Association, hopefully utilising my skills in this area to set up a drop-in centre for struggling students. My experience of studying Medicine also exposed me to the stress of balancing hospital work, a demanding degree course, and an outside life, and I found that in most situations, I thrive under pressure.

During my degree I worked as a nurse, and as a doctor's assistant in therapeutic, surgical and obstetrics departments, and as acting district doctor in out-patient departments of children's medical-prophylactic institutions. These positions required me to put my medical knowledge into practice and involved extensive patient contact in a medical environment. Working as a doctor-intern in the

Scientific Research Institute of Paediatrics in Azerbaijan required me to adapt my skills to a different situation. In the UK, I have been working at Dulwich hospital as a rehabilitation support worker, usually with elderly patients who require a lot of reassurance to rebuild their confidence and who sometimes resist treatment. All of these experiences have shown me that clear and effective communication is essential in developing trust-based relationships between patient and healthcare professional, and that lifelong learning is crucial in retaining expertise in a particular field. I feel that both of these factors transfer well to dentistry, in which empathising with frightened, ill, angry, young or old patients forms part of the daily routine.

Having completed an Art School course, I enjoy drawing and am also a trained pianist and enjoying sewing items for my young daughter. As a DJ in Azerbaijan, hosting a daily live show which featured chat, celebrities and music, I worked with a range of musical equipment such as mixers and CD players, which required considerable dexterity. I also have an interest in languages, being fluent in Russian, English, Turkish and Azeri.

As a mature student I have researched my options thoroughly and am fully committed to training as a dentist. With my background in medicine I know precisely which field I wish to enter and what this work will involve. I am a hard working and extremely well motivated person, and I feel I have the qualities required to succeed at university and in my future career.

Example 21

My interest in dentistry originates from a strong academic background, complemented by pertinent extra-curricular study and relevant work experience. I have a caring and compassionate nature and would like a career that helps others. In 2004/5 I had severe injuries which resulted in my having extensive surgery and time away from school at a crucial time of my exams. Overcoming my injuries and re-sitting my A levels has made me more mature and reflective, and even more determined to become a dentist.

My choice of A level subjects reflects my strong interest in science. Chemistry has given me analytical and practical skills as well as experience of group research. Physics improved my critical thinking skills and in Maths I enjoyed problem solving and methodical calculations. After deciding in my A2 year that I was committed to becoming a dentist I took a double course of AS and A2 Biology in a third year at college.

My interest in science led me naturally to dentistry as a profession and my work placements reflect this. At the age of 16 I arranged a placement at a private practice and observed procedures such as extractions, fillings and cleaning. There was a focus on prevention and I was interested to see the detailed advice the hygienist gave. For the next three years I continued to undertake work experience each summer expanding my knowledge to include implants. At 17 I had braces fitted and I have a positive view of dentistry from a patient's perspective. Resulting from this I have an interest in Orthodontics and may specialise in this area after qualifying. I am also arranging work experience at an NHS practice for comparison and also at a hospital so that I can see the work that Maxillofacial Surgeons do there. Currently, I am working fulltime at Tesco to raise funds for my gap year activities which include a long sailing trip accompanying a group of disabled and underprivileged teenagers. I have applied to Camp America to work there next summer where I will be living with many people of different nationalities and will be looking after children. My gap year should develop me as a person and prepare me well for my future studies.

I relish positions of responsibility, whether as a prefect at school or in my sporting and scouting activities. I am a youth scout leader and look after 10-14 year olds, organising camping trips and teaching life skills. As a successful rugby coach I train an under-16s team. This summer we were selected to tour South Africa after being judged one of the best clubs in England. Training requires empathy, patience and the ability to instil confidence. As a water sports instructor I have extensive interaction with people of all ages which has helped my communication and interpersonal skills. Sailing is my passion and requires excellent teamwork skills to aid health and safety. It also demands a great deal of precision and accuracy together with the manual dexterity required to tie knots quickly and man the sails. At school I played the flute to Grade 5 and took part in the Duke of Edinburgh Award. As a high achiever both academically and in sport, I have excellent time management skills. This, together with all of the above, has given me transferable skills to take to university and to apply to my future career.

I am a highly motivated individual with interests in many areas and a genuine commitment to a career as a dentist. I look forward to making the most of the opportunities available to me at university and having a successful career.

Example 22

My decision to study Dentistry at university is the result of careful consideration and it has required much determination on my part. With a view to studying Dentistry at university, and in order to reinforce the strength of my application, I have gained a number of further qualifications, the most significant of which is a Bachelor of Science. I particularly enjoyed performing dissections on a variety of organisms including frogs and earthworms. These regular practices required manual dexterity to ensure that these procedures were performed carefully and accurately. My enjoyment of this course, and in particular those areas which covered the human body, has confirmed my decision to study Dentistry.

Participating in work experience at a dental surgery has given me an invaluable insight into the day-to-day life of a dentist, and it has fuelled my desire to become one. During my experience I observed many procedures including root canals, fillings and teeth removal. I learnt how to a take a patient's history and along with this, how to empathise with patients in situations that they may find stressful. I plan to build on this work experience with another upcoming placement, something which I have organised myself as a result of my eagerness to learn. Maxillofacial Surgery is something that I am particularly eager to study in greater depth, and it could perhaps offer an area of specialism for me.

Being voted Head Girl was a rewarding but challenging experience. It required me to act as a point of communication between my fellow pupils and teachers, and I was also responsible for the organisation of various events; one such event being a fun fair. I also had to ensure that the school rules were adhered to; this required excellent interpersonal skills in order to communicate my point to fellow pupils. As Head of the Drama Society at school my responsibilities included organising the overall management of productions as well as casting and directing. This required excellent communication skills in order to get the best results from the actors. These skills can only be an asset as a dentist, as it is important to communicate effectively with the patient. It also necessitated good organisational skills: I had to consider all aspects of the production, from arranging rehearsal times to sourcing props. I was also a member of the school debating team and competed in many inter-school competitions. My best performance saw me achieve second place in a regional final and this debating experience has improved my confidence and public speaking skills. My involvement with the Drama Society and debating team was a thoroughly enjoyable experience and something I would hope to continue with at university.

In my spare time I enjoy playing badminton, and I intend to continue this and make full use of the sporting facilities that university can offer me. At school I was a keen member of the cricket and netball teams. My participation in these sports was invaluable in that it has helped me to learn how to work successfully in a team, and it allowed me to make many new friends. I also enjoy glass painting. This has allowed me to develop my artistic ability and also my manual dexterity, something that is essential in dentistry.

While my route to dentistry may not be as conventional as many others, I would hope that my determination and commitment to my future career are unquestionable. This course can help me to fulfil my future career ambitions whilst in the process allowing me to fully develop as a person.

Example 23

Most consumer products in today's world can have damaging effects on oral health which the public may be unaware of. Dentistry allows me to study the methods of prevention and treatment, whilst intricately combining my enjoyment and aptitude for caring and working alongside people. After studying Biomedical Science, I prefer to utilise my knowledge and skill by focusing on a specific subject area.

I find the physiological, immunological and disease aspects of Biomedical Science intriguing, providing an understanding of the human body and diseases. Microbiology lab work has improved my manual dexterity, discipline and organisational skills. Knowledge gained studying Biomedical Science is required in dentistry, which I intend to build and work upon whilst studying. The practical side of dentistry, interaction with patients and carrying out procedures, is what I am looking forward to most. In the future, I would like to open up surgeries of my own to meet demand for dentists. Currently, I am following advances in laser dentistry, as the technology will have a great influence on the future of dental surgery.

To achieve an insight into a dentist's life, I undertook a month's work experience shadowing two practitioners, witnessing procedures such as routine/surgical extractions, root canal treatments and more. During this time, I improved my communication skills through speaking to a diverse mix of patients, allowing me to understand them better. I witnessed an elderly patient, worried about the procedure, and observed how the practitioner handled the situation, explaining the procedure step by step and alleviating her anxiety. Gaining two weeks at a dental laboratory allowed me to see stages in the manufacture of dentures such as Maryland Bridge, increasing my knowledge of dental procedures. This experience and speaking with dentists, showed me there is a significant amount of pressure involved in dentistry and that a calm attitude, time management, attention to detail and interpersonal skills are vital.

Outside of my studies I work part-time for the 'Eurotraveller Hotel' as a weekend manager, leading a team of five senior staff. This demanding role has helped the learn how to deal with stressful situations. As a mentor for year 7 students, I assisted in their transition from primary to secondary school, whilst as a Biomedical student representative, I liaise between the biosciences programme board and students, gathering information and suggesting ideas to improve academic life. I qualified in First Aid with St John ambulance service and for the past year have been assisting my grandmother, who was diagnosed with Pemphigus, taking responsibilities in helping with her medication and ongoing weekly treatments, and assisting other patients in the Chemotherapy ward at King's College. Exposure to these environments has significantly improved my interpersonal and disciplinary skills, which are required in studying Dentistry when trying to finish assignments on time, quickly adapting to situations, working as part of a team or independently, and offering patient care in sessions. Through my hobbies in DIY and computing, I have developed excellent manual dexterity. I also enjoy sports, such as football, which I play weekly. To relax I enjoy listening to and editing music.

Whilst studying Dentistry, I would like to liaise between staff and students providing ideas and methods for improving student academic life at university. Combining the skills I have developed through my experiences, my ambition to succeed in healthcare and my personality as a friendly, confident person and efficient team player, I believe I possess the qualities necessary to pursue a career in dentistry.

Example 24

Dentistry offers me the opportunity to unite my interest in science and technology. I am attracted to the challenges of providing a high standard of patient care and managing a practice effectively. My initial interest was sparked by treatment that I had to align my jaw and straighten my teeth. Since then, I have been fascinated by orthodontic treatments and their effects on a patient's overall well being.

During a work experience placement, I observed dentists perform endodontic treatments which encouraged my ambitions towards the profession and gave me a more in-depth understanding of a dentistry practice. I was also intrigued by the large numbers of different filling materials and composite resins used for filling in cavities, and I look forward to studying more about which materials are used where and why. I am currently undertaking more work experience at a local practice where I am shadowing the dentist during his appointments, as well as performing reception and administrative duties. I am planning to experience NHS and private clinics, as well as completing a work placement in a hospital. My time spent alongside the dentists and dental nurses has allowed me to discover the complexity and importance of oral health and hygiene whilst I also appreciated the need for dentists to persevere with patients and the stamina required for what can be a very demanding role. By expanding my knowledge, I hope to gain a greater understanding of the status of modern dental clinics in the UK.

During my gap year, I plan to return to Tamil Nadu, India, to work in a rural village volunteering in educational and construction projects. Previously, I volunteered by forming play groups at the local school, participated in restoration work at the local temple, and helped to repaint some buildings at the school. I have also helped out in the farms lending a hand during irrigation and harvest periods. Additionally, I have been involved in charitable work for Cancer Research UK and Mind, as well as volunteering with the Winged Fellowship Trust. This has all been rewarding work and has significantly developed my communication skills. I am keen to continue to develop my relationships with these organisations whilst at university.

I am an active and outgoing individual with the ability to stay calm under pressure. My experience within the Combined Cadet Force (CCF) has fostered in me a determination to succeed and a high attention to detail. As a Senior Cadet, I accompanied cadets on exercises and led field trips and generally acted as a mentor to them. I also obtained a First Diploma in Public Services, and had the opportunity to practise my skills and knowledge at the prestigious Frimley Park Cadet Leadership Course. I have also completed my Duke of Edinburgh Bronze and Silver awards and am on course to achieve my Gold.

I have a wide range of extra-curricular activities, and believe that this contributes towards achieving a balanced outlook in life. I participate in rock climbing, kickboxing, hockey, cricket and baseball. I also enjoy playing the guitar. However, my main passion is horticulture, and I recently had the privilege of working with some very skilled and acknowledged gardeners at the Royal Botanic Gardens at Kew. Once at university, I hope to join several clubs and societies, particularly the University Officer Training Corps where I hope to excel to a high level.

In conclusion, I consider myself to be a well-rounded student, with significant relevant experience, and I look forward to the challenges and rewards of life as a dental student and subsequent dentist.

Example 25

My ambition is to pursue a career as a hygiene therapist as it would combine my interest in the promotion of oral health with the opportunity to work in a skilful and creative way with my hands. Having day-to-day contact with a wide range of people appeals to me greatly, as does working within a team of professionals to run a successful business in the community.

As a qualified dental nurse for the past five years, I have learnt about the role and requirements of the hygiene therapist, and the need for skills such as patience and compassion, particularly when attending to nervous patients. Stamina is also required for dealing with large numbers of patients. My experience has included several fields of dentistry, particularly clinical, and I have had the opportunity to work within a dental team alongside hygiene therapists, assisting and observing their work on many occasions. Most of my work involves nursing for Periodontal Surgery and I believe this experience will be very useful for putting the theory I will learn on this course into context, and for preparing me for the clinical practice components of the course.

In my work I interact with many different patients every day, giving me the communication skills that are vital for a hygiene therapist to deliver oral health messages to people of all ages and levels of understanding. Whilst studying on my Oral Health Education course I developed my interpersonal skills by learning to educate people in different ways and I found helping the public to focus on their oral hygiene very rewarding. In my own time I have also been voluntarily giving oral health talks within the Vietnamese community. This has helped to give me confidence in my ability to deliver oral health education to large groups and I am looking forward to building on this during the two weeks of work experience I will complete as part of the course. Becoming more closely involved with treating patients, particularly children and the disabled, is very appealing to me and I am also excited about gaining the expertise required to perform minor extractions and fillings. As well as discussing careers options with my colleagues, I have enjoyed learning more about the opportunities allied to dentistry through the Dental Nursing Association newsletter and other periodicals. Completing my Oral Health Education qualification has been a stimulating return to study and I am also currently retaking my Human Biology and English Literature GCSEs in order to meet the requirements of entry to the course.

In my leisure team I enjoy a range of artistic pursuits such as painting in acrylics, oils and watercolours and sketching landscapes and portraits. I also play both violin and piano and I believe this dexterity will be a useful skill for my future career, for example when cleaning the patient's dentition with hand scalers. In the future I envisage myself having a long career within the NHS and I am particularly hoping to specialise in helping people with disabilities to improve their oral hygiene. I am aware that this course is both physically and mentally challenging but I feel fully prepared for committing myself to the necessary hard work and I look forward to the challenge of achieving success both as a student and in my future career as a hygiene therapist.

Example 26

Two years ago, I attended a careers exhibition arranged by several French universities which presented a series of lectures on potential career paths for students. Having already learned the value of good dental health from a young age, I was especially impressed by the lecture on dentistry. The ways in which a dentist can influence and help a patient are so varied that I knew immediately this was the career I wanted to pursue. It also helped that my favourite subjects at school have always been Science and Maths. In addition, from a young age I have made greetings cards, which I now make and sell to my family. Some of the cards I make are very intricate and require good manual dexterity; a skill I know is essential to becoming a dentist.

Emigrating to France at the age of twelve posed a number of personal challenges; with little knowledge of the language, I had to adapt quickly. Nine-hour school days, including Saturday mornings, required adjustment to a new, demanding schedule. However, I feel that my results reflect not only my academic ability but also my ability to thrive under such pressure. At the age of 15 I took the French equivalent of GCSEs and received the highest grade of 'Tres Bien', awarded for an average, over all subjects, of 80% – and to only seven students in my school. Currently, I am studying for the Science Baccalaureate (a three year course). One module of this measures a student's ability to work on a science project in a small team. The team of students is left totally to their own devices to produce the necessary work/ information for the exam; I took the exam this year and achieved 98%.

My recent placements at two dental surgeries in England have enabled me to observe a wide range of treatments including restorative procedures, Prosthodontics, Endodontics, Periodontics and Orthodontics. Seeing a patient who had been fitted with a brace particularly fascinated me, and the 'before' and 'after' models of her teeth showed me the amazing results such a procedure can produce. I enjoyed interacting with the patients and working within a multidisciplinary team and have arranged another placement for October at Warrington Hospital, where I will have the opportunity to observe surgical procedures.

I am a keen athlete, qualifying for the French National Cross Country Championships and the French National Athletics Championships two years in a row. This year I achieved 6th place in the 1500m, a performance I am particularly proud of. I was also honoured to captain my school athletics team in the Schools National Championships. To achieve this level of attainment, my training regime requires a great deal of dedication and perseverance. Although the events in athletics are mainly individually based it is important that we all work together as a team, training in small groups and supporting each other throughout the season.

As a conscientious and motivated person, I am keen to help others; I have a personal interest in cystic fibrosis and have been heavily involved in fundraising, taking part in sponsored bike rides, bed pushes and 'Stepathons'. This is something I would love to continue at university. I feel that I would make a significant contribution to university life and am certain that both my academic and life experiences have more than prepared me for degree-level studies. I have set my heart on becoming a dentist, and will do everything possible to achieve my goal. As such, I look forward to building on my existing abilities through successfully completing a Dentistry degree.

Example 27

Dentistry appeals as a career because it combines manual dexterity with the practical application of scientific knowledge, and the opportunity to make a positive difference to people's lives. My college studies have given me a secure foundation in science and I have found learning about the functions of the human body in Biology particularly interesting. Chemistry has given me experience of both independent and group research which will be useful for my degree. I have been a hard working and enthusiastic college student and will apply the same commitment to university.

Through a work placement within a dental practice I gained a thorough understanding of the daily workload of a dentist and was able to observe a variety of conditions and treatments. I observed that much of the dentist's work was independent and to tight deadlines, and that the ability to remain calm under pressure was essential when performing delicate procedures. Having decided from this experience that I definitely wanted to work in dentistry, I recently arranged a further placement there. I made the most of this second opportunity to discuss career issues with the staff, and learnt about the managerial skills involved in running a practice. As a naturally sociable person I enjoyed communicating with the range of people I met there, from dental professionals and support staff to patients and their families. At a master class at Liverpool Dental Hospital it was exciting to see the phantom head room and learn more about the structure of the training programmes.

My job as a sales assistant has required consistently high levels of customer service. It is important to adopt a confident and respectful manner, and to remain calm and positive with difficult customers. It is also important not to take such incidents personally. Assisting at The Friday Club for the past two years, I have provided friendship and support for people with special needs and I also volunteered at sports days at a special needs school. At Scouts I have increased my independence and self-reliance through regular camping trips away from home. As a trained Eucharist Minister, my main duties are in assisting with the administration of communion, and such an active role within the Church requires me to communicate with people of all ages with self-assurance.

At school I am a Senior Prefect, which involves supervising a team of other prefects and assisting staff with the smooth running of the school, demonstrating leadership and managerial skills and commitment to the school community. I am also part of the Editorial team which produces the annual school magazine, helping to improve my written communication. As Chairman of the Warhammer Club, I have employed organisational skills and indulged my passion of several years for constructing and painting miniature models. This is an intricately detailed activity requiring a high level of manual dexterity. For relaxation I enjoy playing the double bass and have been awarded several certificates for my swimming, including 'Water Safety and Pool Rescue'. At university I am looking forward to learning basic medical science and developing strong communication skills to aid effective diagnosis and treatment. As I like to express my creativity through complex manual work, I anticipate enjoying restorative surgery and perhaps specialising in Orthodontics.

In working as a dentist I will have the opportunity to serve my community and apply my scientific knowledge to practical situations. I am a highly motivated student and feel that I have the qualities required to succeed at university and in my future career.

Example 28

Since a young age, I have been interested in science and pursuing a science-based career which is proactive and involves working with people. I come from a hard working family of business people and healthcare professionals and have gained lots of useful experience which has helped prepare me to study Dentistry at university level. I am a confident, reliable and responsible person and I truly feel that I have the necessary qualities to become a good dentist.

Being focused on my long term goal from an early age has allowed me to prepare myself both academically and also mentally for the challenges ahead. I have achieved consistently high grades throughout school and college in subject areas which are directly related to dentistry, particularly Science and Maths. I have won several bronze UK Mathematical challenge awards. These subjects have allowed me to develop important analytical and problem solving skills. In addition to my strong academic achievements I have also made special effort to see first hand how a dental practice works and how a dentist goes about their everyday tasks, through shadowing a private healthcare dentist for two weeks. I observed many procedures including the following: fillings, bridges, veneers, and crowning. I also had the opportunity to talk to a dentist who specialised in Periodontics, which I found fascinating.

In order to develop leadership, team-working and communication skills I have made special effort to take on roles of responsibility and help others. I mentor younger students in Science and Maths, as well as supervising a club called 'Lab Rats' where I am responsible for looking after younger students who enjoy scientific experiments. This is something I would like to continue as a university student if given the opportunity. I also volunteer at a charity shop called 'Freshwinds' and have worked as a volunteer for Oxfam as part of my Duke of Edinburgh programme, for which I have a bronze award. These experiences have taught me useful life skills such as the ability to listen, teamwork and leadership.

Looking ahead to studying at university, I am very excited about further developing my knowledge of Biology and Chemistry and getting a deeper understanding of these subjects as they are applied to dentistry. I feel I am suited to studying Dentistry and being a dentist as I enjoy working with people and I can concentrate for long periods. I am also a naturally caring person and always want to achieve the highest possible standards. Dentistry also requires a level of manual dexterity and this is another strength I have. I am good at art, sewing, computer maintenance and home economics. I am aware that the course will be demanding and stressful at times, however, I feel I am well prepared for the challenge and have a lot of outside interests to help me to relax. I play tennis, read books and enjoy attending functions in the local community, such as fund raising events. My long term goal is to become a dental surgeon and work in a dental practice helping patients to build their self esteem through oral health.

To sum up, I have worked very hard in order to study Dentistry at university. I have researched the subject well, gaining an in-depth understanding of the profession. I truly feel that I have the academic and personal qualities required to do well on the course as well as become an active member of the student community. I am looking forward to the challenge and eventually fulfilling my dream in my chosen career as a dentist.

Example 29

Dentistry combines elements of science, technology and the personal skill of the practitioner, and I am drawn to a career which will be exciting, challenging and continuously developing. My passion for the scientific and for helping others is my motivation for studying Dentistry, and I feel that it is a field in which I can thrive.

My work experience within the Belle View and Leeds Road Dental Practices has enabled me to gain an insight into the running of a dental practice. Shadowing the dentists and nurses, I was able to appreciate the adaptability required when presented with a wide range of procedures and diseases, from root canals, denture adjustments and tooth extraction, to gingivitis and periodontitis. I also got the opportunity to carry out a filling, learnt the main stages of the scale and polish process and used the scaler. As part of my ongoing commitment to dentistry, I have organised further work experience at a dental laboratory, an orthodontic clinic and at the 'U Dentistry' cosmetic practice, where they specialise in cosmetic/restorative dentistry, smile rejuvenation, implants and anti-wrinkle treatments.

My work experiences have highlighted the importance of bi-manual dexterity, a skill which I have acquired through building and restoring bikes and model making. The precision and co-ordination required for both hobbies has necessitated the development of using tools with both hands in confined spaces, as well as artistic ability. I gained an awareness of the differences between NHS and private sector dentistry, as well as the necessity of adhering to strict administrative, ethical and confidentiality guidelines within a practice. I was very interested in finding out what the dentists thought about the new NHS reforms and whether they were likely to improve working conditions and availability of treatments to patients within the community. This focus on community is incredibly important to me. I am actively involved in charity and community projects and currently volunteer at a local charity shop; Sue Ryder Care. I am also a member of St John Ambulance, and Vinspired, a school voluntary organisation within the community. Additionally, I volunteer at my local club as a squash coach for juniors, and I run for Comic Relief each year at my local tennis and squash club, raising in excess of £500. Through these experiences, I have gained excellent communication, teamwork and leadership skills, all essential skills for a dentist.

My competitive, focussed and adaptable nature has been developed through playing national level squash, sponsored by Karakal, Fudge and OHS, as well as representing Yorkshire for two consecutive years. I also play county level golf and tennis, alongside, when possible, football, badminton, basketball and swimming. My sporting achievements have instilled in me a natural leadership style, excellent teamwork, and the ability to succeed under extreme pressure. As a member of the school council during years 10 and 11, I developed these time management and organisational skills further through organising events and sharing views with my fellow students. This, alongside my ability to work in a team with people at various levels (students, teachers and heads of year), will stand me in good stead at university.

In addition, I am also in regular paid employment, working the late shift within a department store. I believe that my ability to juggle my sports, charity and paid work alongside my academic demands demonstrates that I am an organised and disciplined individual who is keen to contribute wholeheartedly and enthusiastically in all aspects of my life. It is with this same positive attitude that I am looking forward to embarking on this next step towards reaching my career ambitions of working as a dentist and one day running my own practice.

Example 30

Dentistry combines two of my greatest passions in life: the knowledge and complexity of science, and the skill and dexterity of art. Whilst delving further into the subject I came to appreciate the true satisfaction and variety it brings as a career. It must be very rewarding to enrich a person's life, whether through treating a painful tooth or boosting their confidence with a new smile. Dentistry is the career for me as it is a hands-on profession where I will be able to have a direct impact on patients' lives.

I was fortunate enough to experience a wide array of dental scenarios during my various placements. I have had the opportunity to observe treatments ranging from simple fillings and root canal treatments to complicated crown and bridgework. My placements enabled me to encounter patients from all walks of life and with varying degrees of dental knowledge. This highlighted to me the difficulties in trying to provide the best quality of care, whilst trying to meet the patient's needs, wants and affordability. New advancements such as digital radiography can be especially beneficial in these circumstances as the problem is visualised and the reason for treatment can be fully explained with the use of instant x-rays. I was fortunate enough to witness the placement of two dental implants into the maxilla. This treatment was fascinating as I was able to see the highly developed skill set needed to carry out such a delicate procedure. Work with a local orthodontist and in an Oral Surgery department at a hospital has further broadened my understanding of and experience in the field of dentistry.

Attending a taster course allowed me to gain hands-on experience of preparing fillings and fixing braces onto a set of false teeth. I have also been able to gain some direct experience of working in general practice as a receptionist and assisting the dentist during treatment. I understand that the day-to-day practice of dentistry is a multidisciplinary affair; both leadership qualities and the ability to work as a team are attributes that I possess and continue to develop through the Community Sports Leadership Award and Duke of Edinburgh Bronze and Silver awards. Assisting a year 1 class helped me learn how to break down complex problems into straightforward terms for an easier understanding. I also undertake weekly volunteering at a charity shop where my interpersonal skills have been further developed.

I hugely enjoy my A level subjects. Mathematics and Chemistry have made me proficient at problem solving and lateral thinking. Biology has always fascinated me, and teaches me to be inquisitive about the world. Various science magazines give me a wider knowledge of these subjects. AS level Art provides me with the manual dexterity vital to dentistry. I also enjoy participating in charity events by taking part in the annual 5km Women's Run, and organising events, most recently a Murder Mystery Night where I was responsible for costumes and decoration. I am a keen dancer, and often perform at charity events and large venues such as Trafalgar Square, where I took part in a Guinness World Record. Being a part of the Amnesty International club also gives me the opportunity to raise awareness within my school.

Aside from the necessary communicative and teamwork skills, I believe I have another quality which is necessary to be an excellent dentist: compassion. My genuine compassion for others and their well being is the driving force in my pursuit for a career in dentistry. This is demonstrated by visits to a local nursing home and my charity work. I believe I have the enthusiasm and dedication to pursue what is a demanding yet rewarding career.

Chapter 8

Proofreading your Personal Statement

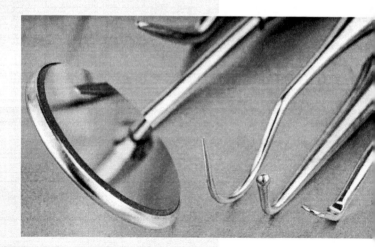

Proofreading your Personal Statement

When you believe that you are ready to submit your Personal Statement, **don't** until you are sure you are happy with its final format. It is also very useful to ask other people to read through your final version; it is amazing how helpful it is to obtain the viewpoint from 'a fresh pair of eyes'. For example, it may be very useful to receive the comments from an English teacher, especially with regard to your punctuation and writing style. Equally, there may be people you met during your work experience who would be pleased to help you in this way. BUT, remember that it is **your** Personal Statement and if you feel passionate about an issue to the point that you are determined to include it, then do so!

Final checklist:

- Do you have a punchy and attention grabbing introduction?
- Do you come over as passionate about studying Dentistry?
- Do you indicate that you have given serious practical consideration to the implications of establishing a dental career for **you**?
- Do you describe how your academic and extra-curricular activities have helped you to make this choice?
- Is every piece of information you provide clearly relevant to your application to study Dentistry?
- Is your Personal Statement arranged in paragraphs? Is it balanced? Does it flow?
- Does your Personal Statement contain a concluding paragraph?
- Check all spelling and all punctuation.

Submitting your Dental School application

The majority of Dental School applications are submitted electronically. Your Personal Statement needs to be typed up electronically and must not exceed 47 lines and 4,000 characters (~580–620 words, size 12 Times New Roman).

If you are applying through your school or college, you will be provided with directions as to how to proceed. Those applying independently, such as graduates or mature students, can register directly on the UCAS website.

For more information visit www.ucas.com

Key points

Keep looking for ways to improve upon your draft effort.

Invite others to proofread your statement before you finally submit it.

Chapter 9

Things to avoid

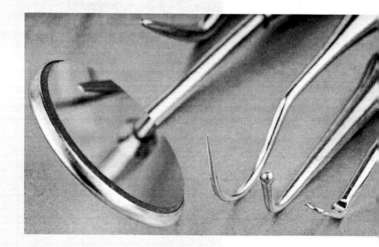

Things to avoid

This guide has focused upon helping you to draft, structure, refine and proofread your Personal Statement.

Here is a list of some things to avoid!

- Rushing the preparation of your Personal Statement – you will need plenty of time to write it!
- Needlessly repeating information that is contained in other parts of your application.
- Relying on a spell checking function – check it yourself; use a dictionary.
- Dishonesty, or deliberately misleading the reader.
- Using any word or phrase the meaning of which you are uncertain.
- Trying to be funny. Just play it straight.
- Drawing attention to any weakness, unless you have learnt from it, handled it, and become a more complete person.
- Including comments which criticise others or casting yourself in a favourable light in comparison to others.
- Simply listing achievements or interests; every comment must be relevant. Lists make for dry reading!
- Disjointed statements. Readers do not like having to flick backwards and forwards when trying to understand your comments.
- Overuse of the 'I' word.
- Lack of structure; lack of paragraphs.
- Not proofreading your statement – ask your teachers, friends and family to help you in this regard. But remember that it is **your** Personal Statement!

Key points

Firstly, always make sure that your Personal Statement really is unique to you.

Secondly, make sure you keep a copy. You can be sure that if you are called for interview, panel members are almost certain to question you specifically upon some of the comments you have made. For you to say 'Oh, I forgot I wrote that' would give an incredibly bleak impression!

Chapter 10

Closing thoughts

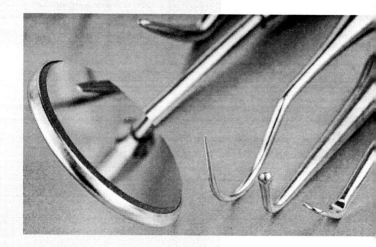

Closing thoughts

The aim of this guide is to provide you with a good idea of what should be included in your Personal Statement for application to Dental Schools in the UK. Our hope is that by following the principles and steps contained in this guide you will be able to compose a well-structured and effective Personal Statement.

For more information on how BPP Learning Media can support you with your application to university please visit:

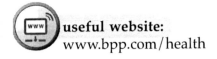 **useful website:**
www.bpp.com/health

We strongly recommend that you do seek more information from Dental School websites, and advice from staff at the Dental School you wish to attend, to ensure that your Personal Statement contains the information that they request.

From all of us at BPP Learning Media we would like to wish you every success in securing your place at Dental School.

Good Luck!!

Appendix

Useful websites

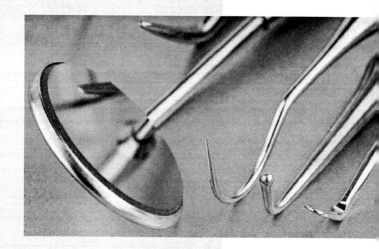

Useful websites

Universities and Colleges Admissions Service
www.ucas.com

General Dental Council
www.gdc-uk.org

British Dental Association
www.bda.org

Dental Schools Council
www.dentalschoolscouncil.ac.uk

United Kingdom Clinical Aptitude Test
www.ukcat.ac.uk